Peripheral Neuropathy

AMERICAN ACADEMY OF NEUROLOGY (AAN)
Quality of Life Guides
Lisa M. Shulman, MD
Series Editor

Alzheimer's Disease
Paul Dash, MD, and Nicole Villemarette-Pittman, PhD

Amyotrophic Lateral Sclerosis
Robert G. Miller, MD, Deborah Gelinas, MD,
and Patricia O'Connor, RN

Epilepsy
Ilo E. Leppik, MD

Guillain-Barré Syndrome
Gareth John Parry, MD, and Joel S. Steinberg, MD

Migraine and Other Headaches
William B. Young, MD, and Stephen D. Silberstein, MD

Restless Legs Syndrome
Mark J. Buchfuhrer, MD, Wayne A. Hening, MD, PhD,
and Clete A. Kushida, MD, PhD

Peripheral Neuropathy
Norman Latov, MD, PhD

Stroke
Louis R. Caplan, MD

Understanding Pain
Harry J. Gould, III, MD, PhD

Peripheral Neuropathy

When the Numbness, Weakness, and Pain Won't Stop

NORMAN LATOV, MD, PhD
Professor of Neurology
Weill Medical College of Cornell University
New York, New York

LISA M. SHULMAN, MD
Series Editor
Associate Professor of Neurology
Rosalyn Newman Distinguished Scholar in Parkinson's Disease
Co-Director, Maryland Parkinson's Disease
and Movement Disorders Center
University of Maryland School of Medicine
Baltimore, Maryland

New York

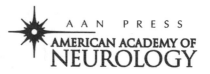

A A N   P R E S S
AMERICAN ACADEMY OF
NEUROLOGY

Demos Medical Publishing LLC, 386 Park Avenue South, New York, New York 10016

Library of Congress Cataloging-in-Publication Data

Latov, Norman.
   Peripheral neuropathy : when the numbness, weakness, and pain won't stop / Norman Latov.
      p. cm. — (American Academy of Neurology (AAN) quality of life guides)
   ISBN-13: 978-1-932603-59-0
   ISBN-10: 1-932603-59-X
   1. Nerves, Peripheral—Diseases—Popular works.   I. Title.
   RC409.L38 2006
   616.8'56—dc22

                                                                    2006020440

Special discounts on bulk quantities of Demos Medical Publishing books are available to corporations, professional associations, pharmaceutical companies, health care organizations, and other qualifying groups. For details, please contact:

Special Sales Department
Demos Medical Publishing
386 Park Avenue South, Suite 301
New York, NY 10016
Phone: 800-532-8663, 212-683-0072
Fax: 212-683-0118
Email: orderdept@demosmedpub.com

Made in the United States of America

09 10 11 12   10 9 8 7

Dedication

This book is dedicated to the memory of Mary Ann Donovan, a dear friend, and founding president of the Neuropathy Association, whose caring, courage, and grace inspired and brought hope to people with neuropathy everywhere.

Contents

About the AAN Press Quality of Life Guides

In the Spirit of the Doctor-Patient Partnership

THE BETTER-INFORMED PATIENT is often able to play a vital role in his or her own care. This is especially the case with neurologic disorders, for which effective management of disease can be promoted—indeed, *enhanced*—through patient education and involvement.

In the spirit of the partnership-in-care between physicians and patients, the American Academy of Neurology Press is pleased to produce a series of "Quality of Life" guides on an array of diseases and ailments that affect the brain and nervous system. The series, produced in partnership with Demos Medical Publishing, answers a number of basic and important questions faced by patients and their families.

Additionally, the authors, most of whom are physicians and all of whom are experts in the areas in which they write, provide a detailed discussion of the disorder, its causes, and the course it may follow. You also find strategies for coping with the disorder and handling a number of nonmedical issues.

The result: As a reader, you will be able to develop a framework for understanding the disease and become better prepared to manage the life changes associated with it.

About the American Academy of Neurology (AAN)

The American Academy of Neurology is the premier organization for neurologists worldwide. In addition to support of educational and scientific advances, the AAN—along with its sister organization, the AAN Foundation—is a strong advocate of public education and a leading supporter of research for breakthroughs in neurologic patient care.

More information on the activities of the AAN is available on our website, www.aan.com. For a better understanding of common disorders of the brain, as well as to learn about people living with these disorders, please turn to the AAN Foundation's website, www.thebrainmatters.org.

ABOUT NEUROLOGY AND NEUROLOGISTS

Neurology is the medical specialty associated with disorders of the brain and central nervous system. Neurologists are medical doctors with specialized training in the diagnosis, treatment, and management of patients suffering from neurologic disease.

Lisa M. Shulman, M.D.
Series Editor
AAN Press Quality of Life Guides

Foreword

NEUROLOGISTS WANT TO HELP patients adjust to—and live with—chronic neurological disease. Peripheral neuropathy is one such condition, which may be caused by many different diseases. One of the most common diseases associated with neuropathy and the current trend of rampant obesity in the United States is diabetes mellitus. However, there are at least 100 other conditions that could lead to neuropathy. Another disease that can lead to neuropathy is Guillain-Barré syndrome, which is a model of those diseases induced by an abnormal immune response. In Guillain-Barré syndrome the patient's immune system attempts to protect the body against infectious bacterium or virus and instead attacks the nerves of the patient. Other so-called "autoimmune" neuropathies are common, and vitamin deficiencies or endocrine diseases are some other factors that can contribute to neurological disease. The word "peripheral" differentiates these conditions from nerves of the brain and spinal cord, which make up the "central nervous system" (CNS). The word "neuropathy" is derived from two Greek words, *neuro* meaning "nerve" and *pathology* meaning the "study of abnormality."

Peripheral neuropathy may be a mild annoyance or a life-threatening condition. Weakness of the legs may cause difficulty in walking and weakness of the hands can interfere with daily functions such as eating and dressing. Sensation can be impaired leading to an abnormal feeling of numbness and tingling. The bladder can be affected and there may be abnormalities of blood pressure or the heartbeat. Each of the component sets of symptoms can be mild or severe. Some are amenable to treatment and some are resistant. It is my hope that patients who read this book would be able to better understand their illness and available forms of treatment.

The chapters in this book follow a logical progression: defining terms, describing the structure of nerves and how their functions can be distorted, defining symptoms, how the diseases are diagnosed, the different causes, and treatment. This information will be useful in helping patients understand the nature of their symptoms, why specific diagnostic tests are done, and what options are available in the treatment of their disease. The patient will feel better informed and, in many cases, will want to take a more active role in plans for treatment with their neurologist. The book culminates with a unique section of stories written by patients themselves, a dose of reality. These stories are told from the perspective of people living with the disease, in the hope that their experiences will be useful to others.

Dr. Norman Latov is an expert on autoimmune neuropathy and all other aspects of neuropathy. He is devoted to helping patients with neuropathy and he was the driving force behind the formation of The Neuropathy Association, an advocacy organization that works to improve care and provides patients with the latest information in the treatment of their disease. This book is another example of Dr. Latov's commitment in helping the patient to gain a better understanding of the diagnosis and treatment of their disease.

Neurologists are physicians who are trained to care for patients with neuropathy. It is therefore fitting that this book is being published as part of a series of books by the American Academy of Neurology that are written by experts and designed for patients, not physicians. This book will be useful in helping the many thousands of people who have incurred various symptoms of neurological disease and provide them with information on the care and treatment of peripheral neuropathy.

Lewis P. Rowland, MD
Professor and Former Chairman of Neurology
Neurological Institute of New York
Columbia University Medical Center
New York Presbyterian Hospital
New York, NY

Preface

IF YOU ARE READING THIS BOOK, chances are that you either have peripheral neuropathy or know someone else who does. Otherwise, you probably would have never heard of it. Although neuropathy is common, estimated to affect 10–20 million people in the United States, most people have never heard of it, and it is difficult to obtain information about the disease.

This book is intended for people with neuropathy, their families or friends, and those who care for them. It reviews what we know about neuropathy, including its causes and manifestations, and what can be done about it. The book also includes stories written by people with neuropathy, who were willing to share their personal struggles with the disease in the hope that their experiences will help others.

Norman Latov, MD, PhD

Peripheral Neuropathy

CHAPTER 1

Introduction: What Is Peripheral Neuropathy?

*P*ERIPHERAL NEUROPATHY REFERS to any affliction of the peripheral nerves. These nerves span the body, similar to wires in an electrical network, and connect the skin, joints, muscles, and internal organs to the brain and spinal cord, which make up the central nervous system. *Peripheral* refers to the fact that these nerves lie outside the central nervous system, so that they are distinguished from central nerves.

The symptoms of neuropathy can vary, but they constitute a limited repertoire. If you talk to ten people with neuropathy, you may hear ten different sets of symptoms, but if you ask another 100, you will probably hear the same ten. The symptoms can be subtle at first, with numbness or tingling in the toes, a sensation as if you are wearing socks and gloves, or that you are walking on sponges or rolled-up socks. You might step on a sharp object or cut yourself, and realize that you do not feel

> If you talk to ten people with neuropathy, you may hear ten different sets of symptoms, but if you ask another 100, you will probably hear the same ten.

any pain. Alternatively, you could experience burning, stinging, or shooting pains in your feet or all over your body, with the pain sometimes so severe that you cannot sleep or think about anything else. Your gait may stiffen and become less fluid, or you might find that your stance is widened or that you tend to lean against a chair or wall when standing, to maintain your balance. Buttoning a shirt, turning a key, or tying your shoelace may become difficult, or your legs might be too weak for you to get up or walk. These seemingly diverse symptoms are all due to peripheral neuropathy. To understand why this is happening, it is necessary to have some understanding what the peripheral nervous system does and how it works.

CHAPTER 2

Function and Organization of the Peripheral Nerves

THREE TYPES OF NERVES: MOTOR, SENSORY, AND AUTONOMIC

THE MANIFESTATIONS OF NEUROPATHY result from disruption of the normal functions of the peripheral nerves. There are three main types of nerves: (1) motor nerves that control muscles and voluntary movement; (2) sensory nerves that transmit signals from specialized receptors in the skin, joints, and internal organs; and (3) autonomic nerves that control involuntary functions such as heart rate, blood pressure, sweating, and the bowel and bladder. Some neuropathies preferentially affect one type of nerve or another, but all three types can be affected to varying degrees, producing a range of symptoms.

STRUCTURE OF THE PERIPHERAL NERVES

The peripheral nerves are made up of *axons*, which are long processes extended from the nerve cell bodies (called *neurons*) that transmit electrical impulses. Motor neurons, which lie in the anterior part of the spinal cord, extend axons that connect to the muscles. Sensory neurons are clustered in sensory ganglia, or collections of neurons, that lie adjacent to the dorsal spine, and extend axons that connect receptors in the skin and joints to other neurons in the dorsal part of the spinal cord. Autonomic neurons lie in autonomic ganglia outside the spinal cord or adjacent to the organs that they innervate. Axons from motor or sensory neurons are bundled in the anterior or dorsal roots as they exit or enter the spinal canal respectively. They then merge with each other and the autonomic fibers as they extend peripherally. Some of these con-

> Different parts of the body are served by different nerves, so that mapping out the sensory and motor deficits sometimes allows the physician to locate the site of injury.

verge in the brachial plexus at the armpit, or the lumbosacral plexus in the pelvis, before fanning out to the arms and legs. Different parts of the body are served by different nerves, so that mapping out the sensory and motor deficits sometimes allows the physician to locate the site of injury.

Nerve axons are further subdivided into small or large fibers. Large fibers are insheathed by an insulating membrane called the *myelin sheath*, which is produced by Schwann cells. The myelin sheath allows for more rapid conduction of the electrical impulse. The large fibers transmit motor signals to the muscles, and sensory signals that convey vibratory sensations or information about the position of joints in space. The small fibers remain unmyelinated; they are slow conducting and transmit signals from pain receptors in the skin. They also form the autonomic fibers that send signals to and from the internal organs. Neuropathies can thereby sometimes be classified as demyelinating or axonal, motor or sensory, small or large fibers, or mixed, and different pathologic processes can cause different types of neuropathy.

PATTERNS OF NEUROPATHY: GENERALIZED, FOCAL, OR MULTIFOCAL

Neuropathies can be generalized, focal, or multifocal. When only a single nerve is involved, usually by focal compression or trauma, the manifestations are restricted to the distribution of that particular nerve.

Examples of focal neuropathy include carpal tunnel syndrome, a condition in which compression of the median nerve at the wrist causes numbness or pain in the palm of the same hand; peroneal palsy, in which compression of the peroneal nerve behind the knee causes foot drop; and lumbar or cervical radiculopathies, in which motor or sensory nerve roots are compressed by a herniated disc or bony spur at the spinal canal.

Some diseases cause discrete lesions that affect some nerves, but spare others, in a multifocal distribution. These are frequently caused by inflammation or infection rather than by metabolic processes that diffusely affect all the nerves. The term *neuronopathy* is used when the neurons, rather than their processes, are primarily affected. *Sensory neuronitis* or *ganglioneuritis* is the term used when the sensory neurons in the dorsal root ganglia are primarily affected. Such processes can also cause deficits in a multifocal distribution as when some neurons or ganglia are affected while others are spared.

The term polyneuritis is used when the neuropathy is generalized, or all the nerves are diffusely involved. This usually causes a symmetric neuropathy that is first manifest in the most distal and vulnerable parts of the body, or the feet and hands. As the neuropathy progresses, the symptoms spread more proximally to the thighs and arms. A common scenario begins with numbness, tingling, or pain in the toes, which then spreads to the ankles and calves in what is called a *stocking* distribution. Since the length of the nerves to the fingers is approximately the same as to the calves, the hands then become similarly affected, in a *glove stocking* distribution. Coordination and balance may become affected as the sensory loss increases. Motor weakness, when it appears, initially affects the distal muscles in the fingers or toes. Weakness of handgrip, as when opening a jar, is an early symptom.

Early involvement of the face is usually indicative of a multifocal neuropathy, neuronopathy, or ganglioneuritis, rather than a distal neuropathy.

Distal, or length-dependent polyneuropathies rarely affect the face or trunk unless the neuropathy is severe, because the nerves to the face or trunk are shorter than the nerves to the limbs. Early involvement of the face is usually indicative of a multifocal neuropathy, neuronopathy, or ganglioneuritis, rather than a distal neuropathy.

SELECTIVE VULNERABILITY: IS IT AXONAL OR DEMYELINATING? LARGE OR SMALL FIBER?

Different pathologic processes can selectively affect distinct anatomical regions or structures of the peripheral nervous system and produce characteristic manifestations. Certain processes can selectively affect the motor, sensory, or autonomic nerves, or primarily the myelin sheaths, axons, or small nerve fibers. Some pathological processes result in a generalized neuropathy, whereas others cause focal or multifocal lesions. Determining the distribution of the neuropathy, the types of nerve fibers that are affected, and whether it is demyelinating or axonal enables the physician to identify the possible causes.

In general, demyelination causes less disability and is more readily reversible than axonal degeneration. However, since myelin and axons are closely intertwined, demyelination can lead to secondary axonal degeneration. Accordingly, in more severe or longstanding cases of demyelinating neuropathy, the neurological deficits are thought to result from irreversible axonal loss rather than the demyelination itself.

Different types of axons can also be selectively affected. Some conditions affect primarily the large axons, resulting in weakness, loss of vibration and position sensations, or incoordination. Others affect the small fibers, and typically cause spontaneous pain with insensitivity to temperature and painful stimuli. The presence of small fiber neuropathy can easily be missed because the electrophysiologic tests, which measure the large fibers, are usually normal. In suspected cases, a skin biopsy may reveal a decrease in the density of small epidermal nerve fibers, confirming the diagnosis of small fiber neuropathy.

CHAPTER 3

Understanding the Symptoms of Peripheral Neuropathy

T HE SYMPTOMS OF NEUROPATHY depend on the type and distribution of the nerves that are affected as well as on the severity of the disease. Early on, the symptoms can be subtle, and they are often ignored or attributed to other conditions such as old age or arthritis. It is important to recognize them, however, so as not to delay diagnoses and treatment. Nerves have a limited capacity to regenerate, and the sooner the condition is diagnosed and treated, the greater the chances the neuropathy can be arrested or reversed before there is significant permanent damage.

MOTOR SYMPTOMS

Motor neuropathy is manifest by weakness in the arms or legs, but early on, the weakness maybe too mild to be recognizable. Subtle symptoms include heaviness in the legs, difficulty getting up from a low chair, pulling on the rail when walking up stairs, or catching a toe on the carpet. The arms may fatigue easily when carrying groceries, or brushing your hair, or turning a lock may require more force. Weakness will become more obvious as the neuropathy progresses. Muscle atrophy or wasting and spontaneous muscle twitching (called *fasciculations*) are also signs of motor nerve damage. Clawing of the toes (called *hammertoes*) is a subtle sign of neuropathy that results from uneven forces pulling on the muscles that flex or extend the toes.

SENSORY SYMPTOMS

Sensory symptoms can be highly variable, and may include pain, insensitivity or loss of sensation (hypesthesia or anaesthesia), spontaneous sensations (paresthesias), unpleasant altered sensations (dysesthesias), or hypersensitivity (hyperalgesia) to pressure or touch.

Pain is normally a protective sensation, providing a warning of existing or pending injury. People who are insensitive to pain may be unaware that they have burned themselves on a hot stove or with hot water; they might step on a nail or another sharp object without feeling any pain. It is not unusual for such people to report that they did not realize they were injured until after they took off their shoes at night and found their foot bloodied.

Paresthesias are variably described as numbness, pins and needles, stinging, prickling, crawling, burning, cold, itching, buzzing, vibrating, aching, tearing, squeezing, stiff, and deadened, or encased in cement, among others. They can occur alone or in combination, and are typically more bothersome at night when there are few other sensory stimuli or distractions, and make it difficult to fall asleep. These symptoms sound bizarre and people who complain of them are often not taken seriously; they may be considered depressed or hysterical by those who are unfamiliar with neuropathy.

Disruption of joint or position sensation prevents the flow of information about the position of the body or limbs in space, resulting in impaired balance or coordination. Symptoms include a widened stance, unsteady or less fluid gait, a tendency to fall, or difficulty with fine manipulations such as tying a shoelace, turning the pages of a book, or buttoning a shirt. The eyes can compensate to some extent by providing visual cues, but balance is rapidly lost in the dark, or in the shower when closing the eyes.

Normal stimuli, such as touch or pressure, can at times cause altered unpleasant or disagreeable sensations called *dysesthesias*. These sensations have variably been described as a feeling of sandpaper rubbing the skin, burning, itching, stinging, ice cold, or lingering, among others. Dysesthesias can be elicited by such ordinary stimuli as light touch or pressure, the feel of clothes against the skin, or a light breeze.

Hypersensitivity to touch or pressure can also cause severe pain, especially in the feet. Tight socks or shoes are particularly a problem, and the pain can make it difficult to walk. Wearing socks without elastic bands, shoes that are soft and roomy, and orthoses that keep pressure off sensitive spots can often bring relief.

AUTONOMIC SYMPTOMS

Autonomic symptoms are less common in generalized neuropathies than sensory or motor symptoms, but they can be the presenting symptoms in predominately autonomic neuropathies. They result from abnormalities in blood pressure, gastrointestinal motility, bladder emptying, sexual functions, temperature regulation, or integrity of the skin.

The autonomic nervous system regulates blood flow to where it is most needed by controlling blood pressure, vascular tone, and heart rate. For example, blood flow is directed to the muscles when running, or to the stomach after eating, which is why it is not a good idea to exercise after a big meal. When standing up from a lying position, the blood vessels in the legs normally constrict to prevent pooling, and the heart pumps a bit faster to ensure sufficient blood flow to the head. In autonomic neuropathy, however, that system fails, resulting in a fall in blood pressure when standing up, a phenomenon that is called *postural hypotension*. The lack of oxygen can cause dizziness or lightheadedness when standing up or, less frequently, headache, neck pain, confusion, or visual blurring. An overly rapid heart beat when standing up (called *postural tachycardia*) can also impair blood flow to the brain.

The autonomic nerves also regulate gastrointestinal motility and bladder emptying. Autonomic neuropathy can cause a lack of physiologic control of the bladder, resulting in atony, loss of bladder sensation, an inability to contract the musculature of the bladder wall, difficulty with initiating a stream, and incomplete bladder emptying, which increases the incidence of infection. There may also be urinary urgency and overflow incontinence. Impaired gastrointestinal motility can cause gastroparesis, with epigastric discomfort or fullness, early satiety, and occasional nausea or vomiting. Bowel dysmotility can cause alternating constipation and diarrhea. Denervation of the internal anal sphincter can cause fecal incontinence.

Autonomic neuropathy also causes sexual dysfunction, manifest by impotence or erectile dysfunction in men, and inadequate lubrication with inability to achieve orgasm in women. Temperature regulation and sweating are also regulated by the autonomic nervous system, and sweating may be impaired in the arms or legs, with compensatory excessive sweating in unaffected areas such as the face or chest. Other manifestations of autonomic neuropathy include swelling at the ankles, dryness and thinning of the skin, hair loss on the legs, delayed healing of the skin, and ridged or brittle nails.

CHAPTER 4

Evaluation
and Diagnosis

Pᴇᴏᴘʟᴇ ᴡɪᴛʜ ɴᴇᴜʀᴏᴘᴀᴛʜʏ can often recognize it in others, as—if in a secret club. One man, for example, was referred to the author after a friend with neuropathy saw him at a party wearing open sneakers with black tie attire. Everyone else thought he was eccentric, but his friend recognized that it was because his feet hurt. Common clues to the

> People with neuropathy can often recognize
> it in others, as if in a secret club.

presence of neuropathy can include reports of bizarre sensations such as tingling or burning, a tendency to lean or keep the feet further apart for balance, taking off shoes whenever possible, such as under the table or when driving, and the presence of hammertoes.

Anyone with symptoms of neuropathy needs to have a neurologic evaluation to see whether, in fact, they have neuropathy, and if so, to find the cause. The neurologist makes a diagnosis of neuropathy based on characteristic symptoms and signs. A detailed history is taken to obtain information about the onset, distribution, and progression of the symptoms, any antecedent events, or coexisting medical conditions and treatments. This is usually followed by a neurologic examination to identify the type, distribution, and severity of any deficits that may be present. Motor functions are evaluated by testing for muscle wasting and strength. Sensory functions are evaluated by testing for perception of pin, light touch, vibration or position in the hands and feet. Balance is tested by standing with the feet together and eyes closed, or walking a straight line, heel to toe. The reflexes at the elbows and knees, which are mediated by both sensory and motor nerves, are also frequently lost in neuropathy. Autonomic function is evaluated by checking for changes in blood pressure and pulse after standing from a lying position. Grading of the deficits in a semi-quantitative manner allows comparisons in subsequent visits to determine whether the neuropathy is stable, improving, or progressing.

Electrodiagnostic tests include nerve conduction studies that determine how the nerves conduct electrical stimuli, and electromyography (EMG) studies that examine the effects of the nerves on the muscles they supply. These tests provide important information about the electrical properties of the nerves, and the type, severity, and distribution of the neuropathy. One important piece of information is whether the neuropathy affects primarily the axons or the myelin sheaths. These studies can be unpleasant, but they are generally well tolerated and helpful in determining the cause of the neuropathy. Quantitative sensory testing (QST), which measures the thresholds at which different sensory stimuli are perceived, are also sometimes done to help quantify and follow the sensory deficits.

Electrodiagnostic studies, however, only measure the large nerve fibers, and provide little information about the state of the small unmyelinated axons. They are typically normal if only the small fibers are affected. To make a diagnosis of small fiber neuropathy, it is necessary to do a skin biopsy with measurement of the density of the epidermal small nerve fibers. A lower than normal nerve fiber density is indicative of neuropathy. The skin biopsy can also reveal loss of epidermal nerve fibers in cases of sensory neuropathy before changes are apparent in the electrodiagnostic studies. The skin biopsy is a relatively benign procedure that is usually performed under local anaesthesia at the ankle and thigh.

If autonomic neuropathy is suspected, the neurologist may also test for variation in heart rate during inspiration and expiration, or order a tilt table test to measure changes in blood pressure and pulse in the supine and and vertical positions. The Quantitative Sudomotor Axon Reflex test (QSART), is another specialized autonomic test that measures the ability of autonomic fibers to stimulate sweating.

In some cases, it is necessary to perform a nerve biopsy in order to obtain tissue for pathologic studies. This may be necessary for diagnosing certain types of neuropathies that are associated with inflammation, abnormal deposits, or pathologic features that cannot otherwise be detected. The sural nerve is often biopsied at the ankle or calf because its only function is to supply sensation to the lateral aspect of the foot—which is left numb after the procedure. Adjacent muscle tissue is often examined at the same time because it sometimes shows the same pathological changes. The nerve biopsy is used sparingly, however, because on occasion it can cause lingering pain. It is therefore only used when the necessary information cannot be obtained by any other means.

A spinal tap is sometimes performed if infection, inflammation, or tumor infiltration of the nerve roots in the spinal canal is suspected. The presence of elevated spinal fluid protein concentration without inflammatory cells is characteristic of certain types of neuropathy such as *Guillain-Barré syndrome* or *chronic inflammatory demyelinating polyneuritis* (CIDP), but this can also be seen in other conditions such as diabetes.

The causes of neuropathy vary, ranging from simple vitamin deficiencies to tumors. Additional blood and urine tests, as well as radiologic studies may be needed in order to identify the cause. The specific tests that will be ordered depend on the type, distribution, and progression of the neuropathy, taking into account such factors as other medical conditions and family history.

The information gathered from the history, examination, and various laboratory tests is then used to decide on the most probable diagnosis. The neuropathy can be classified according to cause, as in diabetic or hereditary neuropathy; according to the manifestations, as in distal or multifocal neuropathy; or according to the underlying pathology, as in small fiber, demyelinating, or vasculitic neuropathy. In approximately one-quarter of patients, however, no cause can be found, in which case the neuropathy is considered to be *idiopathic* (of unknown cause), and the disease is classified only according to its manifestations, as in idiopathic small fiber neuropathy.

The following are some of the terms used to describe the clinical syndromes in patients with neuropathy:

- *Polyneuropathy*—a diffuse neuropathy that affects all the nerves
- *Mononeuropathy*—affects only a single nerve
- *Sensorimotor neuropathy*—affects both sensory and motor fibers
- *Sensory neuropathy*—affects only sensory fibers
- *Motor neuropathy*—affects only motor nerves
- *Distal neuropathy*—affects the most distal parts of the nerves (hands and feet)
- *Proximal neuropathy*—affects the proximal muscles (shoulders or thighs)
- *Small fiber neuropathy*—affects small fiber sensory functions; usually painful
- *Large fiber sensory neuropathy*—affects large fiber sensory functions such as position, vibration, balance, or coordination
- *Multifocal neuropathy*—affects multiple nerves at different sites, but sparing others
- *Autonomic neuropathy*—affects autonomic fibers, causing autonomic dysfunction
- *Lumbosacral plexopathy or amyotrophy*—affects nerves in the lumbosacral plexus, with pain or weakness primarily in the thighs and legs
- *Brachial neuritis*—affects nerves in the brachial plexus, with pain or weakness in the arms
- *Radiculopathy*—affects the anterior or posterior nerve roots as they leave or enter the spinal canal, as in motor radiculopathy or sensory radiculopathy respectively
- *Polyradiculopathy*—affects multiple nerve roots
- *Neuronopathy*—affects the nerve cell body rather than the axon or processes, as in sensory neuronopathy or sensory ganglioneuritis
- *Neuritis*—neuropathy that is caused by an inflammatory condition
- *Demyelinating neuropathy*—primarily affects the myelin sheaths of the peripheral nerves
- *Axonal neuropathy*—primarily affects the nerve axons
- *Ataxia*—unsteady gait
- *Acute onset neuropathy*—Begins suddenly or progresses for up to 6 weeks

- *Chronic neuropathy*—Progresses slowly for more than 3 months
- *Subacute neuropathy*—Somewhere between acute and chronic, progresses for between 6–12 weeks

CHAPTER 5

Causes of Peripheral Neuropathy

IT USED TO BE THAT if you had neuropathy you were presumed to have diabetes or be an alcoholic. Alcoholism was often suspected, for lack of another explanation, and a diagnosis of neuropathy carried a stigma. It was not openly discussed in polite society. Today, we know there are many causes of neuropathy, and although diabetes is probably underdiagnosed, we recognize that alcoholism is an uncommon cause, except in certain high risk individuals.

Diseases that affect the peripheral nerves can have neuropathy as their sole manifestation, or be associated with conditions that also affect other parts of the body. The most common cause of neuropathy in the United

> The most common cause of neuropathy in the United States is diabetes, but in most parts of the undeveloped world it is still leprosy, the same as in biblical times.

States is diabetes, but in most parts of the undeveloped world it is still leprosy, the same as in biblical times. Other causes of neuropathy include metabolic, autoimmune, hereditary, and infectious diseases, as well as tumors, toxins, and drugs. The following is a brief discussion of these conditions.

NEUROPATHY IN DIABETES AND GLUCOSE INTOLERANCE

Diabetes is the most common cause of neuropathy in the United States. There are approximately 16 million people with diabetes in the U.S., with 50 percent having some degree of neuropathy. This includes type I (*insulin dependent*, or *juvenile*, *diabetes*) and type II (*adult onset diabetes*). However, only 20 percent of people with diabetes have symptoms of neuropathy, with the others often unaware that they have it, unless it is

> The likelihood of developing neuropathy and the degree of severity increase with the duration of the diabetes and the increase in blood sugar levels.

identified by their physicians during examination. The likelihood of developing neuropathy and the degree of severity increase with the duration of the diabetes and the increase in blood sugar levels. People who develop neuropathy are also more likely to develop an eye condition called *retinopathy* and a kidney disease called *nephropathy*, which are also complications of diabetes. Nerves have a limited capacity to heal, so it is easier to prevent or stop neuropathy from progressing than to heal it. In early or mild cases, however, neuropathy can be reversed.

The neuropathy seen in diabetes is thought to be caused by multiple mechanisms triggered by high blood glucose levels (called *hyperglycemia*). Consequently, the neuropathy can present in several different ways, depending on which mechanism predominates. One of the effects of hyperglycemia is to alter the metabolism of the nerves, which results in a generalized, distal neuropathy. Another effect is inflammation of the small blood vessels (called *microvasculitis* or *vasculopathy*) that impairs blood flow to the nerves, resulting in small strokes. This can affect a single nerve, causing a focal neuropathy, or involve multiple nerves, causing a multifocal neuropathy. Both mechanisms are active to various degrees in most cases of diabetic neuropathy.

The most common manifestation is that of a generalized, predominately sensory, symmetric polyneuropathy that occurs in approximately 50 percent of cases. Most of the people who are affected have numbness and painful sensations in the feet or hands, but many are not aware of their neuropathy until they step on a sharp object or cut their hand, and then realize they do not feel any pain. Some have a predominately autonomic neuropathy with gastrointestinal symptoms, sexual dysfunction, or dizziness when standing, rather than a distal neuropathy. Autonomic neuropathy can also cause a lack of awareness of low blood sugar levels (called *hypoglycemia*), because the autonomic nerves mediate such changes as heart rate or sweating. Thus, it is important to check blood sugar levels frequently. As neuropathy progresses, there is more sensory loss and the pain may be replaced by numbness, which is easier to tolerate.

Focal and multifocal neuropathies occur less frequently than generalized neuropathy in diabetes, and are probably caused by inflammation or small strokes in the nerves. Common manifestations include Bell's palsy or facial weakness, double vision, radiating pain from the back around the trunk, sciatica-type pain in the leg, weakness in one hand or leg, and foot drop. The nerves of people with diabetes are more susceptible to compression or entrapment, so there is a predisposition to develop carpal tunnel syndrome, which is caused by entrapment of the median nerve at the wrist, as well as other entrapment syndromes. People with diabetes also have impaired immunity, and are more susceptible to developing herpes zoster (also called *shingles*), which can cause a painful neuropathy and skin rash in the distribution of the infected nerves.

Another type of neuropathy that occurs in diabetes is lumbosacral plexopathy (also known as *diabetic amyotrophy*), which presents with pain and progressive weakness primarily in the thighs, and less so in the arms and lower legs. This neuropathy usually stops progressing spontaneously after several months and often improves, with partial or complete recovery. It is frequently preceded by severe weight loss without an apparent cause.

Neuropathy in people with diabetes is common, and people with diabetes who develop neuropathy should also be screened for the other common causes of neuropathy, especially if their neuropathy is not the type that is typically associated with diabetes. Nutritional deficiencies, in particular, should be checked for, especially if there is autonomic neuropathy with gastrointestinal involvement.

Glucose intolerance is a condition in which blood glucose levels can remain high for prolonged periods after eating, but are normal between meals. This is considered a mild form of diabetes or a pre-diabetic state.

> The small fiber neuropathy associated with glucose intolerance is often reversible with diet, exercise, and weight loss.

Studies show that glucose intolerance, by itself, is a common cause of painful small fiber neuropathy, including in cases that were previously thought to be idiopathic, or of unknown causes. Most importantly, the small fiber neuropathy associated with glucose intolerance is often reversible with diet, exercise, and weight loss.

Both type I and type II diabetes mellitus are associated with elevated blood glucose levels, but for different reasons. *Insulin* is a hormone produced by the pancreatic beta cells that lowers blood glucose levels by reducing glucose production in the liver, and by increasing glucose uptake by muscle and fat cells. In type I diabetes, which accounts for 5–10 percent of cases, the pancreatic beta cells that make insulin are destroyed by autoimmune mechanisms. In type II diabetes, which is often associated with obesity, the amount of insulin is either insufficient or the muscle and fat cells become resistant to its effects. Type I diabetes requires treatment with insulin injections; type II diabetes, in early stages, is treated using a diet, exercise and weight loss program that can reverse insulin resistance and reduce the requirement for insulin. If this approach fails, however, patients can be treated with drugs that increase the secretion of insulin, sensitize the cells to its effects, or reduce insulin resistance. In more severe or longstanding cases of type II diabetes, the insulin secreting beta cells can die from exhaustion, in which case treatment with insulin injections is needed.

The presence of diabetes or glucose intolerance is routinely diagnosed by measuring blood glucose levels after an overnight fast. In addition, a glucose tolerance test can be performed 2 hours after consuming a standard drink containing 75 g of glucose. Fasting blood glucose levels of less than 100 mg/dl are considered normal; between 100 and 124 indicate glucose intolerance; and 125 and over are diagnostic of diabetes. In a glucose tolerance test, levels at 2 hours normally remain below 140; levels of 140 to 200 indicate glucose intolerance; and levels above 200 indicate actual diabetes. Another useful measure of diabetes is the hemoglobin A1C test, which measures the amount of glucose chemically bound to hemoglobin. As levels of HgbA1c turn over slowly, the test is an indicator of the average blood glucose levels over many days, rather than at a specific moment in time. Hemoglobin A1c levels are normally below 6.0; higher levels are indicative of diabetes. Any one or all of these measures can be abnormal in the same person.

Although neuropathy is common in both type I and type II diabetes, not everyone with diabetes has neuropathy. Other as yet unknown factors probably contribute to its development. However, if you already have neuropathy, you are obviously more susceptible to developing this complication than someone without neuropathy, and you will need to work harder to control your diabetes. Nerve damage occurs whenever blood glucose levels rise above normal, so it is not sufficient to have a good average. It is important to maintain blood sugar glucose levels in the normal range at all times. You will need to test your levels several times a day, rather than only at the doctor's office, and do whatever it takes—diet and exercise, or medications—to keep your diabetes under control. Maintaining blood glucose levels in the normal range will prevent or delay the progression of neuropathy, as well as the other complications of diabetes, such as kidney and eye disease. Studies show that strict glycemic control reduces the occurrence of diabetic neuropathy by 60 percent over a 10-year period.

Neuropathy, along with vascular disease and impaired immunity, is also a factor in the development of skin ulcerations that can lead to amputation. Atrophy of the foot muscles, with imbalance of toe flexors and extensors, causes loss of the protective muscle over bony surfaces and claw-like deformity of the toes, resulting in increased pressure over the metatarsal heads or bony parts of the feet. Atrophic skin changes resulting from dryness and other autonomic changes can make the skin more susceptible to breakdown and retard healing. Pressure from weight over bony surfaces or ill-fitting shoes can then more easily cause abrasions and ulcerations, or result in the formation of calluses that can become ulcerated. If infection sets in, healing can be further retarded by vascular disease and impaired immunity, and the infection can spread to the bone, causing osteomyelitis. If the infection is not eradicated, gangrene can set in and amputation may be necessary to prevent the spread of infection through the bloodstream to other parts of the body.

Proper foot care is therefore of paramount importance in preventing such complications. People with diabetes should inspect their feet every day, looking for dry skin, cracking, blisters, abrasions, calluses, and early skin ulcers. The feet should be kept clean, washed with mild soap and warm water, and thoroughly dried. Lotions or emollients such as petroleum jelly can be used to prevent drying and cracking. Calluses should be shaved and toenails properly trimmed, and infections should be treated immediately with antibiotics or antifungal agents. Soft shoes that fit properly and lack internal seams, which can put unnecessary pressure on the feet, are also recommended. Shoe inserts and orthoses are useful for distributing pressure evenly under the foot.

Neuropathies Associated with Nutritional Deficiencies and Gastrointestinal Disorders

Vitamin Deficiencies

Deficiencies in vitamins B_1, B_6, B_{12}, and E can cause peripheral neuropathy. Of these, B12 deficiency is the most common, with the others being rare in anyone with a normal diet in the absence of gastrointestinal disease. This is because all vitamins except B_{12} are easily absorbed from the gut, whereas uptake of B_{12} from the gut requires a rather complicated active mechanism that sometimes fails. Deficiencies of all vitamins, however, can result from an inadequate diet, malabsorption, bulimia, or as a consequence of prolonged vomiting, as sometimes occurs in pregnancy. Various gastrointestinal illnesses and bariatric surgery for weight loss can also impair absorption.

Vitamin B_{12} Deficiency

Vitamin B_{12} is abundant in meats, poultry, and eggs. The most common manifestations of B_{12} deficiency are numbness and tingling sensations, with an unsteady gait. Atrophy of the optic nerves with visual loss, or mental changes can also occur. The full syndrome is called *combined systems disease*, which affects the spinal cord, peripheral nerves, optic nerves, and brain. Milder cases can present with a painful small fiber neuropathy. Vitamin B_{12} deficiency can also cause pernicious anemia, which is associated with large red blood cells called *macrocytes*.

Vitamin B_{12} is first released from dietary protein in the stomach by digestion with enzymes that require an acidic environment. The free B_{12} is then bound to a protein called *intrinsic factor*, which is made by parietal cells in the stomach, and the entire complex is actively taken up by receptors in the small intestine. Anything that disrupts this process can cause B_{12} deficiency. For example, reduced stomach acidity sometimes occurs in older people, causing a condition known as *achlorhydria*. Deficiency can also result from excessive antacid use, which can prevent the stomach enzymes from releasing B_{12} from the dietary protein. Deficiency of intrinsic factor can occur as a consequence of autoimmunity, resulting in a condition called *atrophic gastritis* in which there are antibodies to parietal cells and intrinsic factor. Chronic use of metformin in diabetes can also cause B_{12} deficiency. Uptake of the B_{12} complex is also disrupted in some cases of diverticulitis, in various malabsorption syndromes such as celiac disease, or following bariatric surgery that removes or blocks part of the stomach and small intestine. All these conditions can cause B_{12} deficiency.

Diets lacking in meats or eggs, such as vegetarian diets, provide less than the minimal amount of B_{12} needed by the body. Vitamin B_{12} supplements contain crystalline B_{12}, which does not require acid conditions in order to be released, but does require that intrinsic factor and the active uptake mechanism be present. If intrinsic factor is lacking or uptake mechanisms are impaired, B_{12} will have to be taken by injection.

Nitrous oxide (also known as *laughing gas*), which is commonly used in the dentist's office, can bind and inactivate B_{12}. In people with B_{12}

deficiency, inhalation of nitrous oxide can precipitate acute B_{12} deficiency and a severe neurologic syndrome, resulting in damage to the spinal cord, brain, and peripheral nerves.

Deficiencies of B_{12} are diagnosed by measuring blood levels. However, the range of normal is rather large, from 220 to 950, and what is low normal for one person may be too low for another. Most neurologists recommend B_{12} supplementation for levels below 350, because stores at that level can quickly run out. Vitamin B_{12} deficiency can also cause elevation of the enzymes methylmalonic acid and homocysteine, and the diagnosis can be confirmed if these levels are elevated.

Treatment consists of B_{12} supplementation for immediate use and to build up stores. In mild cases, oral supplementation of 1,000 mcg per day can be given because approximately 1 percent is absorbed by passive diffusion. Alternatively, sublingual B_{12}, 400 mcg per day for 2–3 days, can be given in cases of malabsorption. More severe or resistant cases are commonly treated with intramuscular injections of 1 mg of B_{12} per day for 5 days, or 1 mg per week for 10 weeks, and 1 mg per month thereafter. Follow-up blood tests are routinely performed to make sure that normal B_{12} levels are achieved and maintained.

Vitamin B_1 Deficiency

Vitamin B_1 (thiamin) is present in rice, meats, and grains. Thiamine deficiency can cause a condition called *beriberi*, which presents with a painful sensory neuropathy and sensory loss beginning in the feet, followed by generalized weakness, including weakness of the tongue, face, and laryngeal muscles. In some cases, beriberi is associated with edema and heart failure. In the nineteenth century, epidemics of beriberi occurred with the introduction of polished white rice as a dietary staple because stripping of the outer rice hull removed the thiamine. In patients with thiamine deficiency, administration of glucose can precipitate encephalopathy because of the accumulation of lactate from disruption of normal glucose metabolism. Accordingly, comatose patients brought to an emergency room are routinely given thiamine before glucose because of the possibility of thiamine deficiency. Patients deficient in thiamine are advised to take 50–100 mg of thiamine orally per day, with follow-up blood tests to ensure that normal levels are maintained.

Vitamin B$_6$ Deficiency or Toxicity

B$_6$ (pyridoxine) is present in fruits, vegetables and meats. Deficiency of pyridoxine can cause a painful sensory neuropathy, with burning paresthesias in the hands and feet. Conversely, a dietary excess of B$_6$—over 200 mg per day for 6 months or 2 grams daily for 1–2 weeks—can also cause a sensory ganglioneuropathy with large fiber sensory loss. Pyridoxine deficiency can also be caused by INH®, which is used to treat tuberculosis, and by hydralazine in hypertension. Patients taking these drugs, or those who are deficient in pyridoxine, are advised to take pyridoxine supplements of 50–100 mg daily.

Vitamin E Deficiency

Vitamin E is present in vegetable oils and wheat germ. A deficiency of vitamin E causes sensory neuropathy, with ataxia and weakness, and incoordination, as a result of involvement of the dorsal root ganglia and peripheral nerves, spinal cord, and cerebellum. Vitamin E is fat soluble and absorbed from the gut in fats; therefore, diseases that cause fat malabsorption can also cause vitamin E deficiency. This can occur, for example, following bowel resection for Crohn's disease or tumor, or in diseases of the pancreas, because the pancreas secretes the enzymes required to break down fats in the gut. It also occurs in an inherited abnormality affecting fat metabolism called *abetalipoproteinemia*, and in congenital atresia of the biliary duct, which carries pancreatic enzymes to the gut. Vitamin E deficiency can be effectively treated with 1–4 g per day of vitamin E; serum levels can be measured to monitor the patient's response.

Bariatric Surgery

Bariatric surgery is increasingly being used as a means of weight control. There are several procedures employed that either bypass part of the stomach or reduce its capacity, with subsequent weight loss. One to 5 percent of patients develop an acute or subacute axonal neuropathy following the procedure, varying from mild sensory neuropathy to severe sensorimotor neuropathy with weakness and sensory loss. In some cases, this type of neuropathy mimics the amyotrophy seen in diabetes, which is also associated with weight loss. The cause of this neuropathy is not entirely clear. In some cases, it is associated with impaired absorption of essential nutrients such as vitamins or copper, but the procedure also causes various metabolic derangements, including the secretion of insulin, which might contribute to the neuropathy. The incidence of this condition is lower in patients whose nutritional status is carefully monitored following the procedure.

Malabsorption

Malabsorption can occur in patients with various gastrointestinal diseases, depending on severity, including inflammatory bowel diseases, such as celiac sprue and Crohn's disease, or infectious diseases, such as intestinal parasitic infestation and Whipple's disease. The symptoms, in most cases, include significant weight loss, abdominal discomfort or pain, and diarrhea. Occasionally, as in celiac disease, the symptoms may be more subtle, and a high index of suspicion is required to make the diagnosis. Extensive bowel resection for tumor or Crohn's disease can cause various malabsorption syndromes; pancreatitis or pancreatic resection for tumor can result in a deficiency of the enzymes required for absorption of fats and vitamin E. Finally, autonomic neuropathy that affects the gut from causes such as diabetes can impair nutrition, adding to the neuropathy. Treatment of the underlying disease combined with nutritional supplementation is usually effective in ameliorating or arresting the neuropathy.

Celiac Neuropathy

Celiac disease is caused by an allergy to gluten, a protein found in wheat and other grains. This is a relatively common condition, estimated to occur in approximately 1 of 150 people, and although it is not directly inherited, it tends to run in families. The childhood form of celiac disease can come on suddenly and intensely, and be associated with weight loss, diarrhea, and nutritional deficiencies. In milder cases, however, and in approximately 50 percent of adult onset celiac disease, there are minimal or no gastrointestinal symptoms. Treatment of celiac disease consists of eliminating all wheat or grain products from the diet and taking additional vitamin supplements in cases of deficiency.

The neuropathy in most cases of celiac disease is of the small fiber axonal type, and relatively mild, with the diagnosis made by skin biopsy. Some patients, however, develop more severe generalized or multifocal neuropathy with weakness and sensory loss. A predominate autonomic neuropathy can also occur.

The diagnosis is made by screening for antibodies to gliadin, the allergen in gluten, and to tissue transglutaminase, which are elevated in celiac disease. The antibodies may also be mildly elevated in some normal individuals, so that the diagnosis requires confirmation by endoscopy and duodenal biopsy, with pathological studies showing the typical villous atrophy in the duodenal wall.

The mechanism of neuropathy in celiac disease is poorly understood. Some patients improve on a gluten-free diet, but in others the neuropathy first appears while on a gluten-free diet, indicating that other mechanisms, such as autoimmunity, may be involved. Immune therapy can be tried if the neuropathy progresses despite a gluten-free diet and nutritional supplementation.

Alcoholic Neuropathy

Neuropathy used to be common in people with chronic alcoholism because of the combination of alcohol toxicity and nutritional deficiencies, particularly that of thiamine. Social programs and homeless shelters now provide care and proper diet, and neuropathy is much less commonly seen. However, alcohol itself is a neurotoxin that can cause a distal symmetric axonal sensorimotor and autonomic neuropathy, which typically begins with sensory loss and burning or stabbing pains in the legs. Liver enzymes are often elevated due to alcoholic liver damage. In one study, patients consumed a minimum of the equivalent of 100 ml of ethanol per day for 3 years before developing neuropathy. Treatment consists of elimination of alcohol from the diet and correction of any nutritional deficits that might be present. In addition, people with neuropathy from other causes would be well advised to limit or eliminate their alcohol intake because the added insult might aggravate the existing neuropathy.

Ciguatera Poisoning

Ciguatera toxicity results from ingestion of reef fish exposed to a protozoa that produces the ciguatera toxin. Symptoms usually begin with abdominal pain, diarrhea, or nausea several hours after ingestion, followed by paresthesias, including at the lips, dysesthesias, and sometimes weakness. The dysesthesias are sometimes manifest by heat/cold reversal. The symptoms usually abate after a period of several weeks. Cooking the fish does not deactivate the toxin.

Nutrition and Vitamin Supplementation

There is no specific diet that is best for people with neuropathy other than a low carbohydrate diet if diabetes is present, or a gluten-free diet if you have celiac disease. If no specific deficiency is present, then a well-rounded diet should provide all the necessary nutrients you need. Vitamin supplements can be taken, however, to make sure that you obtain the minimum daily requirements, including:

- 100 mg of B_1
- 500 mg of B_{12}
- 50 mg of B_6
- 400 mg of vitamin E
- 5 mg of folic acid

Large amounts of B_6 can *cause* neuropathy, and no more than 50 mg a day should be taken.

AUTOIMMUNE NEUROPATHIES

The function of the immune system is to protect the body from invasion by infectious organisms. It is made up of several types of blood cells, including lymphocytes, neutrophils, and macrophages, which are generated in the spleen, lymph nodes, and bone marrow. The immune system also includes *antibodies*, which are circulating proteins that bind to and damage foreign organisms. Lymphocytes are further divided into B-cells that make antibodies, and T-cells that regulate the immune system and also directly destroy infected cells. Antibodies are divided into three main types; IgG, IgM, and IgA.

Autoimmune disease occurs when the immune system mistakenly attacks the body instead of protecting it. Examples of autoimmune disease include: rheumatoid arthritis, juvenile diabetes, and multiple sclerosis, a disease in which the joints, pancreas, or brain are attacked by antibodies and T-cells respectively. Several types of autoimmune neuropathies have been described. The following is a short list.

Chronic Inflammatory Demyelinating Polyneuropathy (CIDP)

CIDP is a chronic autoimmune neuropathy that targets the myelin sheaths of the peripheral nerves. It is considered chronic because it progresses for more than 3 months, and inflammatory and demyelinating because pathological studies of the affected nerves show inflammatory cellular infiltrates and destruction of Schwann cells and the myelin sheaths. In more severe cases, there is also loss of large axons, probably because of inflammation or loss of trophic factors elaborated by Schwann cells. The reason for development of autoimmunity in CIDP is not known. CIDP is different from multiple sclerosis, which targets myelin in the central nervous system or the brain. Central and peripheral myelin is significantly different, and overlap between the two diseases is rare.

The classical presentation of CIDP in approximately half of the cases includes symmetric, proximal, and distal weakness, with loss of sensation in the arms and legs. Early on, there may be difficulty with such functions as getting up from a low chair, walking up stairs, carrying groceries, or turning a key. The large myelinated sensory fibers that mediate vibration and position are affected more than the unmyelinated small fibers that mediate pain, and although numbness is common, painful paresthesias are less frequent or severe than in the axonal neuropathies. Progression is variable: weakness can progress steadily, be intermittent with stops and starts, or occasionally remit or relapse after several months.

Less typical presentations are more difficult to recognize. In some cases, CIDP causes a distal, symmetric, predominately sensory neuropathy with large fiber sensory loss. Early symptoms in such cases include a widened unsteady gait, incoordination, and numbness or vibratory sensation in the hands and feet. Distal weakness can follow in the ankles and hands as the neuropathy progresses. Another atypical presentation is that of asymmetric sensorimotor neuropathy, with weakness or sensory loss in multifocal distribution. The atypical cases are more difficult to diagnose. Similar presentations can be caused by other types of neuropathy, and a high index of suspicion is needed to make the diagnosis.

There is no specific blood test for CIDP. The diagnosis is made based on the clinical presentation, demonstration of demyelinating changes in the peripheral nerves by electrodiagnostic studies or nerve biopsy, and consideration of other possible causes for the demyelinating neuropathy.

Electrodiagnostic studies, including nerve conduction testing, are particularly useful in CIDP. In addition to establishing the presence of neuropathy, they can show the characteristic changes of slowing, dispersion, or conduction block resulting from stripping or destruction of the myelin sheaths. It is important that these studies be performed by physicians who are expert in their use; otherwise the diagnosis might be missed.

On occasion, the diagnosis is made on the basis of a nerve biopsy examination, which can show evidence of demyelination or remyelination. Biopsy is particularly useful in atypical cases in which electrodiagnostic testing is less definitive. These investigations, however, may require highly specialized pathological studies, including examination of teased nerve fibers. Ideally, the biopsy specimen should be sent to a center where this is routinely performed. Biopsy studies, however, are not always definitive, as when the particular segment examined is not involved in the disease.

Spinal fluid protein concentration is typically elevated in over 90 percent of patients with classical CIDP, but in less the 50 percent of patients with atypical presentations. A spinal tap that shows elevated protein concentration is therefore supportive of the diagnosis of CIDP, but the absence of elevated protein levels does not rule out the diagnosis, especially in atypical cases.

Other causes of demyelinating neuropathy that can mimic CIDP include hereditary demyelinating neuropathy and osteosclerotic myeloma, and should be considered in making the diagnosis. Several drugs, including amiodarone and procainamide (FK 506®), can also be associated with a demyelinating neuropathy similar to CIDP. Other conditions that can be associated with CIDP include nonmalignant IgG or IgM monoclonal gammopathy, hepatitis C infection, Sjögren's syndrome, and ulcerative colitis or Crohn's disease.

Proven therapies for CIDP include intravenous gammaglobulins, plasmapheresis, or corticosteroids. They are each effective in a majority of patients, although some people who do not respond to one may respond to another. These therapies differ in their mechanisms and side effects, and the decision as to which one to use depends, in part, on the patient's predisposition to developing side effects. In cases that do not respond to the standard therapies, treatment with chemotherapy drugs such as azathioprine or cyclophosphamide or other immunomodulatory medications, has been reported to be effective.

Intravenous gammaglobulin (IVIg) preparations consist of purified IgG extracted from pooled blood obtained from thousands of individuals. This extract is treated to remove any infectious organisms and given intravenously over a period of several hours at a time. It is thought to work by preventing the immune system from attacking the nerves. A standard loading dose of 2 g/kg is usually administered over several days, depending on tolerance and convenience. This is followed by booster doses of 0.5 to 1 g/kg every 2 weeks, or 1 to 2/kg every month, for a total of 2–3 months, at which time the neuropathy is reevaluated. Improvement may be seen at 2 weeks to 3 months after beginning therapy, but if there is no improvement in 2–3 months, the IVIG is discontinued. Therapy is continued until there is maximal improvement, and then discontinued or tapered to see if it is still needed. In approximately one-third of cases, the disease is monophasic and the improvement persists. In the other two-thirds, however, the disease relapses and maintenance therapy is needed. The dose is then adjusted as needed.

IVIg treatments are generally well tolerated. A minority of people may develop transient symptoms during the infusions, including muscle aches, headaches, or abdominal discomfort, which can be prevented by reducing the rate of infusion or pre-treatment with Tylenol®, Benadryl®, or Solu-Cortef®. More serious side effects, that can prevent treatment, occur in 1 to 5 percent of cases and include severe allergic skin rash or severe headaches, particularly in people with a history of migraines. The skin rash is treated with topical or systemic corticosteroids and the headache with pain medications. Preparations of IVIg that allow subcutaneous infusion at the abdomen rather than directly into the vein may be better tolerated, although the infusions take considerably longer. Severe side effects are rare, and affect less than one in several hundred people. They include: (1) formation of blood clots in the legs, or other parts of the body particularly in people who are predisposed to clotting; and (2) renal failure in people with preexisting kidney disease who are treated with preparations that contain sucrose.

Plasmapheresis is a type of blood exchange that removes from circulation the antibodies that attack the nerves. It is usually done in a hospital outpatient facility, such as the blood bank, as it requires specialized equipment. Circulating blood is removed from a vein by a machine that separates the plasma from the blood cells. The plasma, which contains the autoantibodies and other proteins, is then discarded, and the cells are returned to the body diluted in artificial plasma. A typical course of therapy consists of 4–5 cycles of plasmapheresis treatments within a period of 2 weeks. If improvement is observed within 2 weeks after the last treatment, maintenance therapy can then be instituted with repeat treatments at intervals of 2–4 weeks, as needed. This therapy is relatively safe, except in people with low blood pressure and those taking ACE inhibitors for hypertension, who can develop episodes of severe low blood pressure. The use of plasmapheresis may be limited by the requirement for veins that can accommodate the larger than normal plasmapheresis catheter. In some cases, a shunt is put in, although that can predispose to infections.

The longest-standing therapy for CIDP is treatment with corticosteroids such as prednisone. These are equally as effective as IVIg or plasmapheresis, but have more severe long-term side effects, including diabetes, weight gain, hypertension, heart disease, osteoporosis, bony fractures, necrosis of the hip, immunosuppression, infections, and psychiatric changes. Thus, neurologists prefer not to use corticosteroids long-term unless the other established therapies are ineffective, poorly tolerated, or unavailable. Therapy is typically initiated at 60 or 80 mg per day orally, and continued for up to 6 weeks. If improvement is observed, the medication is continued until it plateaus, at which point it can be slowly tapered to the smallest dose that is still effective. Alternate day oral therapy or intravenous therapy for several days per month can be used to reduce the chances of developing adverse effects. Corticosteroid medications cannot be stopped abruptly after being taken for more than 10 days because they cause the adrenal glands to stop making endogenous steroids such as adrenaline. Stopping the medication abruptly causes a deficiency of adrenaline, in which case the body can go into shock, especially if there is stress or infection. Slowly tapering the medication allows the adrenal glands to resume normal function.

Chemotherapy agents such as azathioprine (Imuran®) or cyclophosphamide (Cytoxan®) are also sometimes used in cases in which the standard treatments are ineffective or cannot be tolerated. These agents, which kill rapidly dividing cancer cells, are also used for immunosuppression because they kill the rapidly dividing T- and B-cells in autoimmune diseases. Chemotherapy agents have more severe side effects, so they are not used as the first line of therapy. Azathioprine can cause abdominal pain, bone marrow suppression, or secondary tumors in a small number of cases. Cyclophosphamide use is associated with secondary malignancies, bone marrow suppression, or hepatic, lung, or cardiac toxicity in a minority of cases. In CIDP that is unresponsive to any of these agents, other immunomudulatory drugs or even bone marrow ablation have been reported to be successful in some cases.

Multifocal Motor Neuropathy and Multifocal Demyelinating Sensorimotor Neuropathy (Lewis Sumner Syndrome)

Multifocal motor neuropathy is an autoimmune condition that attacks primarily the motor nerves in a multifocal distribution. Early on, only the arms may be affected, but it can also affect the legs. This condition often progresses with stops and starts, and causes weakness and muscle atrophy. In approximately half the cases, it is associated with an antibody against GM1 ganglioside, which is present in both myelin and axons in the peripheral nerves. The mainstay therapy is maintenance IVIg treatment, which prevents or slows the progression. This neuropathy does not respond to plasmapheresis, and can be aggravated by corticosteroids. Chemotherapy agents, such as cyclophosphamide, can also be of benefit, but their use is limited because repeated treatments are required and cumulative doses can be toxic.

Multifocal demyelinating sensorimotor neuropathy presents with multifocal weakness and sensory loss in the distribution of individual nerves. It is similar to multifocal motor neuropathy, except for the sensory loss, which also occurs in CIDP. It is also treated with immune therapies such as IVIg.

Neuropathy with IgM monoclonal gammopathy and Anti-MAG or Ganglioside Antibodies

A monoclonal gammopathy occurs when a single clone of antibody secreting B-cells, expands abnormally and secretes antibodies in excess. This condition is called an *IgM monoclonal gammopathy* when the antibodies are of the IgM type. In some of these cases, the monoclonal IgM antibodies are thought to cause neuropathy by binding to antigens, or target molecules in the peripheral nerves. Several different antigens have been identified. In about half the cases, the monoclonal IgM binds to MAG, or the myelin-associated glycoprotein; in others, they bind to other molecules called *gangliosides* or *sulfatide*.

The neuropathies that are associated with the IgM monoclonal gammopathies are typically slowly progressive, and depend on the distribution of the target antigen. IgM anti-MAG antibodies bind to myelin and cause a distal demyelinating polyneuropathy. Those that react with GM1 or GD1a gangliosides are associated with a predominately motor neuropathy, whereas those that are directed at GD1b gangliosides or sulfatide are associated with distal sensory neuropathy. IgM anti-GM1 antibodies also occur in some cases of multifocal motor neuropathy, in the absence of a monoclonal gammopathy. In all these instances, the IgM antibodies recognize the carbohydrate or sugar molecules that are associated with lipids or protein in peripheral nerve. IgG antibodies, which react with some of the same antigens, are associated with more acute or rapidly progressive neuropathies, as in Guillain-Barré syndrome and variants.

IgM monoclonal gammopathies are detected by a test called *serum protein immunofixation electrophoresis*, in which the serum proteins are separated on a gel by an electric field. They are then further characterized by testing for binding to a panel of target antigens. The B-cells that secrete the monoclonal IgMs are akin to a benign tumor, because although they divide more rapidly than normal cells, they are not usually malignant. In approximately 30 percent of cases, however, they can progress to a B-cell malignancy, including to Waldenstrom's macroglobulinemia, or B-cell leukemia, or lymphoma. It is therefore recommended that everyone with an IgM monoclonal gammopathy undergo a bone marrow biopsy to make sure that the gammopathy is not malignant. As progression to malignancy occurs at a rate of approximately 1 percent per year, it is recommended that the bone marrow biopsy be repeated every few years.

Treatment is directed at lowering the concentration of the monoclonal IgMs by killing the B-cells that secrete them. The antibodies can also be removed by plasmapheresis, which is helpful in some cases, but in most people the antibodies rapidly re-accumulate, and treatments are needed too frequently. IVIg is only of limited benefit, mostly in people with weakness. Increasingly, the first line of therapy is rituximab, a therapeutic monoclonal antibody that reacts with, and kills B-cells. A typical treatment consists of four intravenous infusions at 1-week intervals, which is then repeated every 6 months. If rituximab is insufficient, then a chemotherapeutic drug that is effective against B-cells, usually fludarabine, is added. These two drugs are thought to have additive effects, and the combination is thought to be more effective than either drug alone. The response to therapy is monitored by neurologic examination and by measuring the serum IgM levels. After the IgM is lowered with rituximab and fludarabine, lower IgM levels can often be maintained with rituximab therapy alone. There is no cure for this condition, but the aim of therapy is to keep the monoclonal IgM concentrations low. This limits the damage and allows the nerves to heal.

Autoimmune Sensory Neuronitis (Ganglioneuritis)

Autoimmune sensory neuronitis, or sensory ganglioneuritis, results from inflammation of the sensory neurons in the sensory or dorsal root ganglia. The inflammation is usually spotty, and the resulting neuropathy is typically multifocal, rather than distal and symmetric. Symptoms can occur in any part of the body, including the limbs, trunk, or face. It can affect small or large fibers, and cause pain, loss of sensation, incoordination, or gait instability. It can progress steadily or with starts and stops, and varies from mildly annoying to severly painful, and debilitating.

Ganglioneuritis is sometimes associated with Sjögren's syndrome, which is a rheumatologic condition that also causes dry eyes and mouth due to inflammation of the salivary ducts in the mouth and the lacrimal glands in the eye. The neuropathy may affect all sensory modalities or present as a small fiber neuropathy. Sjögren's syndrome can also be associated with vasculitis, and involve the joints, mucosal membranes, or brain. Blood tests often show the presence of elevated anti-SSA-Ro and SSB-La antibodies. Other tests for ganglioneuritis include the Schirmer test, which consists of placing strips of paper in the lower conjunctiva to measure tear production, or instilling rose Bengal dye, which is taken up in damaged areas in the cornea or conjunctiva. A salivary gland biopsy at the lip can confirm the diagnosis, even in cases in which the blood tests are negative. Sjögren's syndrome is usually treated with corticosteroids or azathioprine.

In rare cases, sensory ganglioneuritis is associated with lung cancer. In these cases, the immune system attacks a protein in the cancer cells called *Hu*, which is also present in the sensory neurons and nerves. The neuropathy affects all sensory modalities, particularly vibration and position, and causes incoordination and gait instability. This condition is usually associated with weight loss. A blood test can reveal the presence of anti-HU antibodies. Lung cancer can be identified by chest X-ray or CT scan, and treatment consists of chemotherapy. In rare cases, the neuropathy can be arrested by chemotherapy, even if the cancer is not found, presumably as the result of eradication of the cancer cells.

People who present with a clinical picture of sensory ganglioneuritis are therefore routinely tested for the presence of Sjögren's syndrome and lung cancer. In such cases, identification and treatment of the underlying systemic disease can be lifesaving.

Autoimmune Autonomic Neuropathy

Autonomic neuropathy can also be caused by autoimmune mechanisms. It can be diagnosed by testing for anti-ganglionic acetylcholine receptor antibodies. The most common symptoms are those of orthostatic hypotension or gastrointestinal dysmotility. In some cases, it is associated with cancer. It can be treated with plasmapheresis or intravenous gammaglobulins.

Vasculitic Neuropathy

Vasculitic neuropathy is caused by inflammation of the blood vessels in the peripheral nerves. Destruction of the blood vessels prevents flow of oxygen and nutrients, and causes small strokes along the length of the nerves. The inflammation can be generalized or spotty, and the neuropathy can be either multifocal or diffuse, affecting both motor and sensory fibers, with multifocal or symmetric weakness, pain, or sensory loss.

When the vasculitis is non-systemic or only affects the nerves, the diagnosis is often difficult to make. A nerve and muscle biopsy is usually required to see the pathological changes of inflammation in the blood vessels. This diagnosis is suspected in anyone presenting with multifocal neuropathy of otherwise unknown cause, although some cases present with a distal and symmetric neuropathy, which has no distinguishing features. A nerve and muscle biopsy may therefore be recommended in cases of progressive neuropathy of unknown etiology, because it could be caused by vasculitis.

Other organs in the body, besides the peripheral nerves, can also be affected in systemic vasculitis. Such cases can be diagnosed on the basis of systemic manifestations, such as a skin rash, involvement of the joints, kidneys or lungs, intermittent fevers, or abnormal blood tests. In some cases, the vasculitis is associated with rheumatologic or connective tissue diseases, such as rheumatoid arthritis, lupus, or Sjögren's syndrome. In other cases, it might be induced by an allergic reaction to drugs. Table 5-1 lists the more common systemic vasculitis syndromes that cause neuropathy.

Vasculitic neuropathy is usually treated with prednisone and either oral or intravenous cyclophosphamide, a chemotherapeutic agent. Other chemotherapeutic agents, such as oral azathioprine or intravenous methotrexate, can be substituted for cyclophosphamide. Treatment is required for several months until the disease is quiescent, and the medication is then slowly tapered over 6–12 months. Vasculitis can be a life-threatening disease and leave permanent damage; therefore, early diagnosis and treatment are important.

Guillain-Barré Syndrome and Variants

Guillain-Barré syndrome is a demyelinating polyneuropathy that begins acutely, progresses for up to 6 weeks, and then spontaneously remits. The severity varies, ranging from mild weakness to total paralysis, including of the respiratory and facial muscles. More severe cases are cared for in the intensive care unit, where patients can be closely monitored and provided with supportive care to maintain respiration and

Table 5-1 Common Systemic Vasculitis Syndromes that Cause Neuropathy

Syndrome	Presentation	Other Organ Involvement	Abnormal Laboratory Tests
Polyarteritis Nodosa	Multifocal, distal	Skin, kidneys, testicles, bowel	ESR, rheumatoid factor, hepatitis C, cryoglobulins
Churg-Strauss syndrome	Multifocal, distal	Asthma, sinusitis, skin, kidneys	ESR, eosinophilia, ANCA
Wegener's granulomatosus	Multifocal, distal	Lungs, sinusitis, uveitis, skin	ESR, ANCA, rheumatoid factor
Temporal arteritis	Multifocal, distal	Headaches, muscle and joint pains, eyes	ESR, rheumatoid factor
Sjögren's syndrome	Multifocal, distal, ganglioneuritis, small fiber	Dry eyes and mouth, skin rash, arthritis, Raynaud's syndrome	SSA-Ro and SSB-La antibodies, ESR, ANA
Systemic sclerosis	Multifocal, distal, small fiber esophagus	Fibrotic skin changes with calcium deposits,	ANA, anti-centromere antibodies

blood pressure, prevent bed sores, contractures, or blood clots, and treat infections or irregular heart rhythm during the period of vulnerability.

The disease is caused by inflammation and destruction of the myelin sheaths of the peripheral nerves by the immune system. It can follow or be triggered by events that disrupt normal immune regulation, such as infection, vaccination, surgery, or trauma. Most patients make a complete or nearly complete recovery over a period of months to a year, but some are left with significant residual motor or sensory deficits. The disease is fatal in approximately 10 percent of cases, usually from complication such as infection, pulmonary embolism, or arrhythmia during the acute illness. Other than supportive care, therapy includes plasmapheresis, which removes the circulating antibodies that attack the nerves, or intravenous gammaglobulins, which inhibit the immune attack. Both of these therapies have been shown to shorten the duration of the progressive phase of the disease and hasten recovery.

The classical syndrome begins acutely and targets the myelin sheaths of the motor and sensory nerves. It causes a diffuse demyelinating polyneuropathy, with weakness and sensory loss in the arms and legs. There are also variants that target other parts of the peripheral nerves, including: (1) acute motor axonal neuropathy (AMAN), which presents with weakness and targets the axons of motor nerves; (2) Miller-Fisher syndrome (MFS), which presents with double vision and gait instability resulting from damage to the extraocular and sensory nerves; (3) acute sensory neuropathy that targets the sensory nerves; and (4) acute autonomic neuropathy, in which the autonomic fibers are preferentially involved.

Patients with Guillain-Barré syndrome or its variants frequently exhibit high titers of IgG antibodies to gangliosides, which are complex molecules made up of fatty acids and sugars that are highly concentrated in the peripheral nerves. AMAN, in particular, is associated with antibodies to GM1 or GD1a, and MFS is associated with antibodies to the ganglioside GQ1b. GBS and its variants may therefore be caused by immune reactivity to gangliosides. Other studies have shown that the intestinal pathogen *Campylobacter jejuni* (Cj) is a frequent trigger of AMAN or MFS, and that it contains molecules called *lipopolysaccharides* (LPS), which resemble the gangliosides GM1, GD1a, or GQ1b. It is therefore thought that immune reactivity to the LPS contained in Cj results in development of anti-ganglioside antibodies, which also attack the nerves. The mechanism by which immune reactivity to an infectious organism triggers an autoimmune disease is referred to as *molecular mimicry*.

Proven treatments for GBS include intravenous gammaglobulins or plasmapheresis (see previous section on CIDP). Treatment with intravenous gammaglobulins is generally preferred, because GBS can be associated with autonomic instability, with a predisposition to developing hypotension as a consequence of the fluid shifts that may occur during plasmapheresis.

NEUROPATHIES CAUSED BY INFECTIONS

Viruses, bacteria, parasites, and other infectious organisms can directly infect the nerves and cause peripheral neuropathy.

Virus Infections

Herpes Zoster (Shingles) and Cytomegalovirus (CMV) Infections

Herpesviruses are present in the dorsal root ganglia sensory neurons of most normal individuals since in childhood. These viruses are normally latent or suppressed, but they occasionally become active. Eruption of Herpes simplex viruses are responsible for cold sores and genital herpes. The herpes zoster virus causes shingles, a painful nerve infection, which typically presents as a vesicular rash and pain along the distribution of the infected nerve, in a belt-like pattern around the trunk, or in the limbs or face. The vesicular eruption usually begins to crust and heal after about a week, but in a significant number of cases, the pain continues after healing, in which case it is called *post-herpetic neuralgia*. Occasionally, in more severe cases, the motor fibers in the same nerves are also affected by inflammation, and weakness occurs. Shingles is more common in older or immunosuppressed individuals, in whom it can also be more severe.

Early detection and treatment with the antiviral agent, Acyclovir®, or a related medication can limit infection and the subsequent nerve damage, reducing the severity of the disease. Post-herpetic neuralgia is treated topically with Lidoderm® patches, or with systemic medications for neuropathic pain.

Cytomegalovirus is another herpesvirus that causes neuropathy; it is also a rare cause of acute inflammatory polyneuropathy, or Guillain-Barré syndrome. This virus is more common in patients being treated with immunosuppressive agents following organ transplantation, or in people with AIDS.

Hepatitis C Infection

The hepatitis C virus, which infects the liver, is also associated with peripheral neuropathy. In most cases, this neuropathy is thought to be caused by inflammation of the blood vessels in the peripheral nerves, or vasculitis, resulting from deposits of hepatitis C virus and antivirus antibodies in the blood vessel walls. In some cases, the complexes precipitate in the cold, forming a substance called *cryoglobulins*.

Less commonly, hepatitis C infection is associated with chronic inflammatory demyelinating polyneuritis (CIDP), which is caused by autoimmune mechanisms. In these cases, the virus is thought to trigger the disease by stimulating the immune system.

The vasculitic neuropathy associated with hepatitis C is usually treated with antiviral agents. CIDP, in addition, is also treated with intravenous gammaglobulins. Steroids are also sometimes used but may reduce immunity to the virus. Use of plasmapheresis is limited by the formation of cryoglobulins.

HIV-I Infection

This virus is most commonly associated with a painful sensory or small fiber neuropathy. Several mechanisms are thought to be responsible, including inflammatory mediators secreted by infected immune cells in the peripheral nerves, direct infection of sensory ganglia cells with the virus, and certain antiviral drugs that cause nerve toxicity. The painful small fiber neuropathy associated with HIV-1 infection is usually treated symptomatically with drugs that reduce neuropathic pain.

HIV-1 infection is less commonly associated with several other types of neuropathy. A disease similar to Guillain-Barré syndrome can occur early in the course of HIV-1, or at the time of initial infection. Some people develop a vasculitic neuropathy with inflammation or infection of the blood vessels. Infection of the nerves with herpes zoster virus or cytomegalovirus occurs more frequently in AIDS as the result of immunosuppression. Treatment consists of anti-HIV-1 drugs plus IVIg or plasmapheresis for Guillain-Barré syndrome or vasculitis, and antiviral agents for the herpesvirus.

Peripheral Neuropathy in Lyme Disease

Lyme disease is caused by a spirochete called *Borrelia burgdorferi,* which is transmitted by the bite of a tick. In about half of the cases, the infection is associated with a typical skin lesion that spreads from the site of the bite, forming a reddish patch or target with clearing at the center. During the weeks following the infection, the organism may disseminate to other parts of the body, causing fatigue, malaise, fevers, chills, headaches, or stiff neck. The lesion, which is called *erythema migrans,* and the systemic symptoms occur only in approximately half of the cases. There may be no warning signs in some patients.

Neuropathy can occur after dissemination or in the later stages of the disease. During the weeks to months after infection, it can present with a mononeuropathy such as facial palsy, multifocal neuropathy or polyradiculoneuritis, or distal symmetric neuropathy. It can also present with Guillain-Barré syndrome, or evidence for meningitis with inflammatory cells in the spinal fluid. Cardiac disease or arthritis may also be present at the same time.

Treatment with antibiotics at this stage of the illness eradicates the disease in most cases, but some people have persistent symptoms or exacerbations, which are thought to be the result of irreversible nerve damage, persistent low grade infection, or development of autoimmunity. The neuropathy in such cases can be multifocal, distal and symmetric, or small fiber, with evidence for axonal degeneration. Other manifestations of chronic Lyme disease include arthritis and neuropsychiatric disease with cognitive changes, which may be present in addition to the neuropathy.

Diagnosis of the primary infection is relatively straightforward if the typical skin lesion is present. In its absence, however, the primary infection can be missed, and subsequent diagnosis is based on presence of an immune response, with demonstration of antibodies specific to *B. burgdorferi* by laboratory testing. Blood is typically screened for antibodies using the *Enzyme Linked Immunosorbent Assay* system (ELISA), in which an extract of *B. burgdorferi* is coated onto plastic wells, the serum is added, and the binding of serum antibodies to the extract is measured. If the serum demonstrates higher binding than is seen in normal individuals, it is then tested further by a more specific assay called *Western blot*, wherein the major protein of the *B. burgdorferi* proteins are separated, so that reactivity of antibodies to each of the proteins can be examined. Antibodies of the IgM class appear first, with IgG antibodies only appearing later. Thus, the presence of IgM, but not IgG, antibodies to *B. burgdorferi* signifies a recent infection.

There is quite a bit of debate regarding the reliability of these types of assays, because the diagnosis depends on demonstration of antibodies, rather than the infective organism. Antibodies to *B. burgdorferi* may not appear for several weeks after infection, or the response could be blunted in immunocompromised or partly-treated individuals. False positives may occasionally be seen in the ELISA system, particularly in people with other inflammatory or immune diseases; antibodies to some of the *B. burgdorferi* protein bands can be present by Western blot in some normal individuals. In general, the more sensitive assays have a higher rate of false positivity, but the less sensitive it is, the higher the chance of false negatives or missing the diagnosis. In most cases, however, the assays are quite reliable.

Some laboratories offer assays based on new technology called *polymerase chain reaction* (PCR). They can detect DNA sequences of *B. Burgdorferi* in tissue, blood, or urine. These assays are also subject to false positives and negatives, and there is no consensus as to their reliability.

Therapy early in the disease with oral doxycycline 100 mg twice a day, or amoxicillin 500 mg four times a day, for 10 days to 2 weeks is recommended for erythema migrans to eradicate the spirochete and prevent the later complications. For later stages, when neuropathy or other neurologic disease is present, treatment with intravenous ceftriaxone, 2 g per day for 4 weeks, or with oral doxycycline, 100 mg a day for 4 weeks, is recommended. Treatment with 100 mg twice a day of oral minocycline, which is related to doxycycline, is also sometimes used because it is concentrated in neural tissue.

Neuropathy Caused by Bacterial Infection: Diphtheric Neuropathy

Diphtheric neuropathy is rare in developed countries with preventative childhood vaccination. It still occurs, however, in less economically privileged areas. The neuropathy is caused by a toxin that is elaborated by the bacteria, and is similar to Guillain-Barré syndrome in that it progresses for several weeks and then spontaneously remits. The illness typically begins with a throat infection that is characterized by formation of a grayish-white exudate, or membrane, that adheres to the underlying mucosa. The neuropathy begins at 3–4 weeks into the illness, initially with paralysis of the throat and facial muscles, followed by generalized weakness and sensory loss in the arms and legs. Recovery begins after days to weeks. Infections can also occur at other sites, including the skin. The diagnosis is made by bacterial culture and typing. Treatment with anti-toxin within 48 hours reduces the severity of the neuropathy and limits the illness. Supportive therapy is given during the period of paralysis to maintain respiration, nutrition, and cardiovascular functions. The childhood DPT vaccine induces antibodies to the diphtheria toxin, providing long-lasting immunity to the illness.

Sarcoid Neuropathy

Sarcoid is a disease that is characterized by the presence of granulomas, which are collections of inflammatory cells in various tissues. It is thought to be caused by an infectious agent, although the causative agent has not been identified. Sarcoid neuropathy can present as a mononeuropathy with facial nerve palsy, mononeuritis multiplex, distal and symmetric sensorimotor neuropathy, or as small fiber neuropathy. It is thought to be due to the presence of granulomas in the peripheral nerves.

The diagnosis of sarcoid neuropathy may be difficult to make if the disease is confined to the peripheral nerves without involvement of other organs. When other organs are involved, such as in pulmonary or skin sarcoid, biopsy of one of the lesions can confirm the diagnosis. This condition is sometimes associated with elevated calcium or immunoglobulin levels, which, if present, can provide a clue and lead to the diagnosis.

Otherwise, a high index of suspicion is required to prompt the physician to order a nerve and muscle biopsy, which may reveal the presence of the granulomas. Sarcoid neuropathy is usually responsive to corticosteroids.

Neuropathies Caused by Parasitic Infection: Chagas' Disease

Infection with *Trypanosoma cruzi* causes Chagas' disease, which is the most common infectious disease in Central and South America. The infection causes inflammation and destruction of nerve cells in both the peripheral and central nervous systems, as well as of muscle cells, with cardiomyopathy, and enlargement of the hollow muscular organs such as the colon or esophagus. The neuropathy is generalized or multifocal, with significant autonomic involvement. Chagas' disease is transmitted by insects, through discharged feces, and can enter the body through contaminated food, blood, broken skin, or mucosal membranes.

LEPROSY

Leprosy is a chronic disease of the peripheral nerves that is caused by infection with *Mycobacterium leprae*. The disease is rarely fatal, but can cause serious disfiguration and disability. Because of the disfigurement and fear of contagion, people with leprosy have been shunned or segregated in leprosarium since biblical times, although modern medications and views have changed this more recently. Leprosy, however, remains the most common cause of neuropathy in undeveloped countries.

Mycobacterium leprae is an intracellular organism that lives inside the Schwann cells, which are the myelin forming cells of the peripheral nerves. It has a predilection for the cooler parts of the body, such as the earlobes, elbows, knees, nose, and tips of the fingers or toes. The neuropathy is usually associated with raised skin lesions of various sizes or shapes that are insensitive to pain or other sensory stimuli. In one form of the disease, referred to as *tuberculoid leprosy*, the skin lesions are well localized, sharply demarcated, often hypopigmented, slowly enlarging, and have a reddish border. In the more disseminated lepromatous form, the lesions are more varied in size or shape. Biopsy studies of the skin lesions usually reveal the presence of *Mycobacterium leprae*, confirming the diagnosis. The deformities are largely due to the skin lesions and loss of protective sensation with repeat injuries, particularly of colder parts of the body, such as the hands, feet, and face. Blindness can occur as a consequence of invasion of the eyes.

The neuropathy of leprosy is characterized by sensory loss, which is often noticed after suffering an injury without feeling any pain. On examination, there is loss of pin and temperature sensations, with relative preservation of vibration or position, which probably indicates damage to the cutaneous nerves. In the tuberculoid form of leprosy, the sensory loss occurs in patches, in the region of the skin lesion, with enlargement of adjacent nerve trunks. These result from infiltration of inflammatory cells in response to the infection. The sensory loss is distal and symmetric in lepromatous leprosy, and in a glove stocking distribution, which then spreads more proximally. As the disease progresses, the motor fibers of the more superficial nerves, such as the ulnar nerves or facial nerves, also become affected, resulting in multifocal weakness in addition to the sensory loss.

Leprosy is treated with a combination of medications, including dapsone, rifampin, and clofazimine. Improvement is slow, and occurs over months or years.

NEUROPATHY IN CANCER AND LYMPHOPROLIFERATIVE DISORDERS

The relation of neuropathy to cancer is complex. Most people with cancer who develop neuropathy have a toxic neuropathy caused by chemotherapy agents. Rarely, the neuropathy is *paraneoplastic*, meaning it is caused by an immune reaction to a protein present in both the tumor cells and the peripheral nerves. In addition, B-cell tumors can secrete autoantibodies that damage peripheral nerves, and herpesviruses can cause infection in people immunosuppressed by chemotherapeutic drugs. Finally, the tumor cells can directly infiltrate or compress the peripheral nerves. All these are mechanisms by which cancer can be associated with peripheral neuropathy.

Neurotoxicity Caused by Chemotherapy and Radiation Sensitizing Agents

Chemotherapeutic agents that can cause neuropathy include vincristine, cisplatin, Taxol®, thalidomide, bortezomib, and related agents. Generally, these drugs cause an axonal neuropathy, although with some differences in their major manifestations. The neuropathy is usually related to the cumulative dose of the chemotherapy, limiting its usefulness. The neurotoxic effect is more severe in people with preexisting neuropathy, and screening for neuropathy is advisable prior to the use of these agents. The following is a list of the anticancer agents that cause neuropathy.

Vincristine and Related Agents

Vincristine is used to treat lymphoma, leukemia, and some solid tumors. It causes a mixed sensorimotor and autonomic neuropathy, with axonal degeneration of both myelinated and non-myelinated fibers. It is dose-related, limiting the amount of drug that can be given. The most common manifestations are painful paresthesias, with sensory loss in the arms and legs, constipation and abdominal pain caused by autonomic neuropathy, and mild distal weakness. The symptoms usually improve within 3 months after the medication is stopped, although residual symptoms may linger. Vincristine is thought to exert its effect by binding to microtubules in the axons, interfering with axonal transport and causing axonal degeneration. There are no known agents that protect against the neurotoxicity, but symptomatic therapy for pain helps while waiting for improvement.

Cisplatin and Related Agents

Cisplatin is used in the treatment of cancers of the lung, ovaries, testis, bladder, colon, and head and neck. It causes neuropathy after cumulative doses of 300–600 mg/m². The neuropathy typically affects large sensory fibers, causing numbness and paresthesias, with impairment of vibration and position, incoordination, and imbalance. The neuropathy may progress for several months after cessation of the drug, a phenomenon referred to as "coasting." The neuropathy then improves slowly over months and years, but often with some permanent residual nerve damage. The mechanism of neurotoxicity is poorly understood, although it is probably mediated by binding to DNA in dorsal root ganglia sensory neurons.

Paclitaxel (Taxol®)

Paclitaxel is used to treat solid tumors of the breast, ovary, lung, and head and neck. It causes a predominant sensory axonal neuropathy.

Approximately 50 percent of the patients who take paclitaxcl gradually develop neuropathy at cumulative doses of greater than 700–1400 mg/m^2, or abruptly after single doses of 300–350 mg/m^2. Typical symptoms include numbness, burning paresthesias, and impairment of all sensory modalities in the hands and feet. In more severe cases, balance and muscle strength can also become affected. Improvement occurs over several months after cessation of the medication, although in more severe cases there may be permanent residual deficits.

Thalidomide

Thalidomide is used in the treatment of multiple myeloma and in several dermatological disorders related to leprosy and autoimmune conditions. Thalidomide causes a distal axonal neuropathy, primarily affecting small fibers, with numbness and painful paresthesias. The neuropathy resolves if the medication is stoppcd soon after appearance of the symptoms, but in more severe cases there may be only partial or no improvement.

Bortezomib

Bortezomib is the first of a new class of agents that inhibit the proteasomes involved in intracellular protein degradation. It is currently used for the treatment of multiple myeloma and non-Hodgkin's lymphoma, but its use is expanding to other tumors. It appears to cause neuropathy in approximately one third of cases.

Misonidazole

Misonidazole is used to sensitize cells before radiation therapy for cancer. It causes a distal axonal neuropathy with burning and lancinating pains in the hands and feet. All sensory modalities are affected. Weakness can also occur in more severe cases. The neuropathy gradually improves after the medication is discontinued.

Paraneoplastic Neuropathy

Paraneoplastic neuropathies are caused by tumors resulting from indirect mechanisms. The best characterized of these is the sensory neuropathy that is associated with cancer of the lung and anti-HU or ANNA-1 antibodies. This causes a progressive sensory neuropathy affecting all sensory modalities, with loss of vibration and position in the hands and feet, resulting in impaired balance and incoordination. There is often weight loss related to the tumor, and in some cases the central nervous system can also be affected. The neuropathy is thought to be caused by immune reactivity to the Hu protein, which is shared by the tumor cells and neurons. Treatment is directed at the primary tumor, with stabilization of the neuropathy in some cases.

Autoimmune autonomic neuropathy with anti-ganglionic acetylcholine receptor antibodies has also been associated with several types of tumor, including of the lung, bladder, rectum, and thyroid. The neuropathy in such cases is manifest by orthostatic hypotension and gastrointestinal dysmotility. The same autoimmune syndrome can also occur in the absence of cancer.

Neuropathy in Myeloma and POEMS Syndrome

Myeloma is a neoplastic disorder of plasma cells in the bone marrow. Plasma cells produce IgG or IgA antibodies, and myeloma is usually associated with the occurrence of monoclonal IgG or IgA antibodies in the blood. In some cases, the same types of monoclonal antibodies occur in the absence of tumor, in association with chronic inflammation or benign proliferation of the plasma cells. The IgG or IgA monoclonal antibodies are different than the IgM monoclonal antibodies secreted by B-cells, and are associated with a different type of neuropathy.

Osteosclerotic myeloma is distinguished from other myelomas by the presence of calcified sclerotic changes on X-rays of the bones or skeletal survey. The presence of myeloma can also be detected or confirmed by a bone marrow biopsy of the involved area. The IgG or IgA antibodies are almost always of the lambda type, as opposed to ordinary myelomas, which can be either lambda or kappa. Approximately 50 percent of osteosclerotic myelomas are associated with peripheral neuropathy, which is frequently demyelinating and may mimic CIDP. It is also sometimes associated with the POEMS syndrome, which includes polyneuropathy, organomegaly with enlarged liver or spleen, endocrinopathy, such as diabetes or thyroid disease, monoclonal gammopathy, and skin changes, including increased pigmentation, thickening of the skin, or white nail beds. Other features include clubbing of the fingers, edema, and increased red blood cells or platelets. POEMS syndrome can occur in the absence of monoclonal gammopathy, in which case the gammopathy is assumed to be present at levels below the limits of detection. Recent studies suggest that POEMS syndrome is due, in part, to secretion of high levels of *vascular endothelial growth factor* (VEGF), in which case it would respond to anti-VEGF agents. Treatment of the underlying myeloma frequently ameliorates the neuropathy.

Some cases of neuropathy associated with osteosclerotic myeloma may initially be misdiagnosed as CIDP, which can also be associated with nonmalignant IgA or IgG monoclonal proteins in the absence of myeloma. However, unlike CIDP, the demyelinating neuropathy associated with osteosclerotic myeloma does not respond to plasmapheresis, IVIg, or corticosteroids, and is almost always associated with the lambda light chain. A lack of response to these agents, or the presence of a lambda light chain or features associated with the POEMS syndrome, should alert the physician to the possible diagnosis of osteosclerotic myeloma.

Neuropathy with Primary Amyloidosis

Amyloid neuropathy is caused by deposition of amyloid in the peripheral nerves. This neuropathy is typically painful, and involves both sensory and autonomic fibers. There are two main types of amyloidosis: hereditary and acquired. In hereditary amyloidosis, the deposits consist of a mutated form of the protein transthyretin, whereas in acquired or primary amyloidosis the deposits consist of fragments of the light chains of monoclonal immunoglobulins, usually IgG or IgA. Primary amyloidosis can be associated with myeloma or B-cell malignancies, as well as monoclonal immunoglobulins secreted by nonmalignant cells. In some cases, only the immunoglobulin light chains are expressed, and because of their small size, they are secreted in the urine where they can be detected by immunofixation electrophoresis or as Bence Jones proteins.

Diagnosis of primary amyloidosis requires demonstration of deposits of amyloid and immunoglobulin light chains in the nerve or other affected organs, such as the skin, abdominal fat, rectal mucosa, or bone marrow. In some cases, the deposits can only be identified by a nerve and muscle biopsy. Amyloidosis is a life-threatening condition, not only because of the neuropathy, but also because of involvement of the heart and other organs. Therapy is directed at eliminating the antibody secreting cells using chemotherapeutic agents, or even bone marrow ablation therapy.

Neuropathy with Waldenstrom's Macroglobulinemia or B-cell Leukemia or Lymphoma

In contrast to plasma cells, which secrete IgG or IgA immunoglobulins, B-cell tumors, including Waldenstrom's macroglobulinemia, chronic B-cell leukemia, and B-cell lymphoma, secrete monoclonal IgMs. In approximately 75 percent of cases, the monoclonal IgM immunoglobulins cause an autoimmune neuropathy by reacting with antigens in peripheral nerve. The specific neuropathic syndromes associated with these antibodies are discussed in the section on autoimmune neuropathies.

Neuropathy Caused by Tumor Infiltration

Focal compression or infiltration of nerve by tumor cells produces deficits in the distribution of the nerves that are infiltrated. Depending on the location or type of tumor, the nerve roots along the spinal cord, the brachial or lumbosacral plexus, or individual nerves, alone or in combination, may be affected. Focal enlargements of the nerves, or compression, may be visualized by MRI scanning.

NEUROPATHY ASSOCIATED WITH RENAL FAILURE

Most people with renal failure (called *uremia*) have some degree of sensorimotor neuropathy. The neuropathy is typically distal and axonal, and presents with numbness, tingling or burning paresthesias, and tenderness in the feet. Restless leg syndrome, with creepy crawling and itching sensations, may also occur. In more advanced cases, there may also be distal weakness in the legs. On examination, large fiber sensory modalities or vibration are affected more than pin and temperature. Treatment is directed at the underlying uremia, with more frequent dialysis or renal transplantation, resulting in improvement or resolution of the neuropathy.

NEUROPATHY ASSOCITED WITH THYROID DISEASE

Neuropathy is common in untreated hypothyroidism, but this rarely occurs nowadays because of early diagnosis and treatment. The neuropathy is predominately sensory and associated with painful distal paresthesias and unsteadiness resulting from large fiber sensory loss. Compressive focal neuropathies, particularly carpal tunnel syndrome, also occur because of thickening of the ligaments and tendons from deposits of a substance called *mucopolysaccharide*. Hypothyroidism can also cause myopathy with proximal weakness in the legs. Treatment of the hypothyroidism results in amelioration of the neuropathy.

HEREDITARY NEUROPATHIES

The hereditary neuropathies compromise a heterogeneous group of diseases. They are caused by mutations or other alterations in genes that directly or indirectly affect the peripheral nerves. Over twenty genes have been identified, to date, as being associated with hereditary neuropathies. The genetic abnormalities can be inherited or occur spontaneously, after which they are passed on to subsequent generations. Inheritance varies, however, with autosomal dominant neuropathies requiring that only one copy of the gene, from either parent, be mutated, whereas autosomal recessive neuropathies require both copies of the gene, one from each parent, to be affected. X-linked disorders result from mutations in the X-chromosome, and they typically occur in men in whom only one X-chromosome is present.

Neuropathics that occur in families with greater frequency than in the overall population can also occur as a consequence of genetic predisposition, rather than direct inheritance; as occurs, for example, in diabetes, celiac disease, and monoclonal gammopathies. Accordingly, the presence of neuropathy in more than one family member, does not necessarily mean that the neuropathy is hereditary, or that it will necessarily occur in future generations. A discernable pattern of inheritance, or demonstration of a DNA mutation that is associated with neuropathy, are necessary to confirm the presence of a hereditary neuropathy.

Traditionally, the hereditary neuropathies were categorized according to the clinical presentation, and whether they were axonal or demyelinating. Two main nomenclatures or classification systems were used interchangeably: one based on *Charcot-Marie-Tooth* disease (CMT), and the other on subtypes of hereditary neuropathy, including *hereditary motor and sensory neuropathy* (HMSN), *distal hereditary motor neuropathy* (dHMN), and *hereditary sensory and autonomic neuropathy* (HSAN). For example, hereditary sensorimotor neuropathies that were demyelinating, or caused by genes expressed in myelin-producing Schwann cells, were classified as subtypes of CMT type 1 or HMSN 1, whereas axonal sensorimotor neuropathies were classified as subtypes of CMT type 2 or HMSN 2. X-linked neuropathies were classified as CMTX. The hereditary demyelinating neuropathies are further subdivided according to their mode of inheritance, with the autosomal dominant neuropathies classified as subtypes of CMT1, and those with autosomal recessive inheritance as subtypes of CMT4.

These clinically based classifications are still useful in most cases, but with the advent of DNA testing, it has become evident that there are many exceptions. Mutations in different genes can cause similar clinical manifestations, and the same or different mutations in the same genes can result in entirely different clinical presentations. Other, as yet unknown factors, appear to affect the clinical manifestations in any one patient. Therefore, genetic testing is increasingly relied on to diagnose and categorize this group of diseases.

The most common type of hereditary neuropathy is CMT1A, which is caused by duplication of PMP22 gene. This type of neuropathy occurs in approximately 70 percent of patients with hereditary demyelinating neuropathies, and in 20–30 percent of all hereditary neuropathies. In its classic form, it presents with a slowly progressive distal sensorimotor neuropathy that begins in the first 2 decades of life, with such symptoms as clumsiness, poor balance, or difficulty running. Most people retain the ability to walk, although ankle supports or aids to ambulation are often required. Some affected individuals do not develop symptoms until adult life. CMT1A is associated with stork legs (atrophy of the calves), pes cavus (high arches), and hammertoes (clawing). The foot deformity is thought to be caused by imbalance, or uneven pulling of opposing foot muscles, secondary to the neuropathy. Deletion of the PMP22 gene is commonly associated with *hereditary neuropathy with predisposition to pressure palsies* (HNPP), which is manifest by episodes of demyelination, with focal weakness and sensory loss. Point mutations in the PMP22 gene can be associated with both the distal and HNPP phenotype. Dejerine-Sottas disease (DSD), also called *HSMNIII*, is a severe demyelinating neuropathy that occurs in infancy, and is associated with point mutations in the PMT22 gene, P0 gene, EGR2 gene, or periaxin.

The most common form CMT2, is CMT2A, which is associated with mutations in MFN2, and presents with a distal axonal neuropathy. It affects approximately 20 percent of patients with CMT2. Many of the other hereditary neuropathies are quite rare.

Hereditary neuralgic amyotrophy is an autosomal dominant recurrent hereditary neuropathy that causes brachial plexitis. It has recently been linked to mutations of a gene encoding Septin 9 (SEPT9).

Peripheral neuropathies also occur in several hereditary diseases with systemic manifestations that affect other organs in addition to the peripheral nerves. In familial amyloid neuropathy, the sensory nerves are primarily involved with pain and prominent autonomic symptoms, including postural hypotension and gastrointestinal irregularities. This neuropathy is caused by mutations in transthyretin, a protein that is secreted by the liver. The mutated transthyretin is deposited in the nerves, heart, kidneys, and intestines. The disorder is life-threatening, but can be treated by liver transplantation because the new liver will secrete normal transthyretin.

Acute intermittent porphyria causes attacks of neuropathy, with abdominal pain and neuropsychiatric manifestations. This neuropathy is often of sudden onset, with weakness and autonomic dysfunction, and may be confused with Guillain-Barré syndrome. It is detected by elevated urine porphyrin levels. Variegated phrphyria is similar, except it also causes a rash. Both are inherited in an autosomal dominant fashion. Attacks can be precipitated by certain drugs, barbiturates in particular, that interfere with the metabolism of porphyrin, an iron binding compound in cells. It is treated by supportive care, particularly for the autonomic symptoms, and may respond to intravenous hematin.

Fabry's disease is an X-linked disorder that occurs in men; it can cause a painful sensory neuropathy, with lancinating or burning pains. Fabry's is associated with a small, raised, reddish skin rash, in a bathing trunk distribution, called *angiokeratosis*. It results from accumulation of glycosphingolipids, and is associated with vascular, heart, and kidney disease.

Mitochondrial neurogastrointestinal encephalomyopathy (MNGIE) is an autosomal recessive disorder caused by a mutation in the gene encoding thymidine phosphorylase. The full-blown syndrome is associated with gastrointestinal disease, central nervous system disease, muscle disease, impairment of eye movement, and sensorimotor neuropathy. It results from impairment of energy production by mitochondria inside the cells. In a small number of cases the initial manifestations may be similar to CIDP.

At the time of this writing, there are no therapies that can prevent the onset or progression of most of the inherited neuropathies. However, physical and occupational therapy can help maintain function, with the help of orthotics and bracing when needed. Occasionally, surgery to correct ankle or foot deformities, such as Charcot joint, pes cavus, or hammertoes, can help improve walking, alleviate pain, and prevent ulcers at pressure points. Genetic counseling can provide advice regarding inheritance and prognosis.

Table 5-2 lists of the primary hereditary neuropathies for which the responsible genes have been identified, along with their mode of inheritance, phenotype, and associated clinical features.

DRUG-INDUCED NEUROPATHIES

Peripheral neuropathy can be caused by drugs that are toxic to the neurons or Schwann cells in the peripheral nerves. In most cases, the neuro-

Table 5-2   Primary Hereditary Neuropathies

Abnormal Gene	Name	Inheritance	Axonal/ Demyelinating	Clinical Manifestations
Peripheral Myelin Protein P2 (PMP22)	CMT1A/ HNPP	AD	D	DS, HNPP, DSD
Myeline PO Protein (MPZ)	CMT1B	AD	D, A	DS, DSD
Simple (LITAF)	CMT1C	AD	D	DS
Early Growth Response Protein 2 (EGR2)	CMT1D	AD	D	DS, DSD
Gap Junction Beta-1-Protein (GJB1)/ Connexin 32	CMTX	X-linked	D	DS
Mitofusion 2 (MFN2)	CMT2A	AD	A	Distal axonal neuropathy
Ras-related Protein Rab 7 (RAB&)	CMT2B	AD	A	Predominately sensory axonal neuropathy
Glucosyl-tRNA Synthetase (GARS)	CMT2D/ dHMN V	AD/AD	A	Sensorimotor or motor neuropathy
Neurofilament Protein, Light Chain (NFL)	CMT2E	AD	A	DS
Heat Shock Protein 27 (HSP27)	CMT2F	AD	A	DS
Ganglioside-induced Differentiation Protein 1 (GDAP1)	CMT4A	AR	A or D (hypo-myelination)	Onset in infancy, severe sensorimotor neuropathy, ± vocal cord paralysis
Myotubularin-related Protein 2 (TMR2)	CMT4B1	AR	D	Infantile onset, sensorimotor, distal and proximal weakness

(continued on next page)

Table 5-2   Primary Hereditary Neuropathies (continued)

Abnormal Gene	Name	Inheritance	Axonal/ Demyelinating	Clinical Manifestations
SET Binding Factor 2	CMT4B2	AR		DS
NDRG1 Protein (NDRG1)	CMT4D	AR	D	DS, deafness
Periaxin (CMT4F)	CMT4F	AR	D	DS, DSD
Heat Shock Protein 22 (HSP22)	dHMNII	AD	A	Motor neuropathy
Serine Palmitoyl-transferase Light Chain 1 (SPTLC1)	HSAN I	AD	A	Small fiber sensory functions are primarily affected, painful and with ulcerations
Hereditary Sensory Neuropathy 2 (HSN2)	HSAN II	AR	A	Early onset, severe sensory neuropathy
1 kappaB Kinase Complex-associated Protein (KBKAP)	HSAN III (Familial dysautonomia, Riley-Day)	AR	A	Infantile onset, autonomic and sensory neuropathy
Tyrosine Kinase for Nerve Growth Factor (NTRK1)	HSAN IV	AR	A	Congenital insensitivity to pain with inability to sweat, overheating
Septin 9 (SEPT9)	HNA	AD	A	Recurrent brachial plexitis

CMT: Charcot-Marie-Tooth disease
HNPP: hereditary neuropathy with predisposition to pressure palsy
dHMN: distal hereditary motor neuropathy
HSAN: hereditary sensory and autonomic neuropathy
HNA: hereditary neuralgic amyotrophy
D: distal neuropathy
HNPP: hereditary neuropathy with predisposition to pressure palsy
DSD: Dejerine Sottas syndrome
AD: autosomal dominant
AR: autosomal recessive
D: demyelinating
A: axonal

pathy is dose-dependent and improves after the medication is discontinued. The effect of these drugs may be more severe in people with pre-existing neuropathy, and they should avoid using these drugs if at all possible. The extent of recovery depends upon the severity of the damage and the regenerative capacity of the nerves. The drugs commonly used for cancer therapy that can cause neuropathy are discussed earlier in this chapter—the following is a discussion of the other commonly used medications that can cause neuropathy.

Amiodarone

Amiodarone is used to treat cardiac arrhythmias. Neuropathy occurs in 6–10 percent of cases, appearing 1½–2½ years after beginning the medication. It causes a demyelinating neuropathy similar to CIDP, with weakness and distal sensory loss. Improvement usually begins several weeks after stopping the medication, and may continue for a year. Recovery may be incomplete in severe cases. Amiodarone is an amphophilic, or lipid binding agent, that is thought to exert its action on the myelin sheaths by forming lipid complexes that are resistant to degradation, and that form inclusions within Schwann cells.

Chloramphenicol

Chloramphenicol is an antibiotic that is rarely used because of its toxicity. It can cause optic neuropathy, sometimes accompanied by peripheral neuropathy, after prolonged treatment over several months. The neuropathy is distal and axonal, and presents with painful burning sensations in the feet. The neuropathy usually resolves completely after discontinuing the drug.

Chloroquine

Chloroquine is used in the treatment of malaria and rheumatologic or connective tissue diseases. It causes a neuromyopathy, with damage to both nerves and muscles, which can occur after several months or years of treatment. It presents with increasing weakness in the limbs, and sometimes in the neck and facial muscles, and occasionally sensory loss. Chloroquine is also an amphophilic agent, and electrodiagnostic studies may show a demyelinating neuropathy in addition to the muscle damage. Improvement occurs over many months after cessation of the medication. Recovery may be incomplete in severe cases.

Colchicine

Colchicine is an antiinflammatory agent that is commonly used for gouty arthritis, and occasionally for other inflammatory conditions. It causes neuropathy and myopathy (muscle disease), mostly in people with renal insufficiency who take the drug for prolonged periods. It usually causes both proximal weakness in the thighs and distal sensory loss. Elevation of the muscle enzyme CPK supports the presence of toxicity. Symptoms usually improve over a period of months after stopping the medication or lowering the dose.

Dapsone

Dapsone is used for the treatment of leprosy and certain dermatologic disorders. The neuropathy is dose-dependent, and occurs in some patients at doses of 200–300 mg/day when used to treat the dermatological disorders, but not at the lower doses used to treat leprosy. It causes a motor neuropathy with distal weakness in the arms and legs, and variable sensory loss. The neuropathy improves following cessation of medication. Extent of recovery depends on the degree of axonal loss.

Disulfiram

Disulfiram is used in the treatment of chronic alcoholism. It can cause a distal axonal neuropathy, with painful burning sensations followed by weakness in the hands and feet. Recovery is incomplete, and the medication should be discontinued as soon as symptoms appear. It should not be taken by people that abuse alchohol who already have neuropathy.

Ethambutol

Ethambutol is used in combination therapy for the treatment of tuberculosis. It can cause optic neuritis, with visual loss, and less commonly a distal predominately sensory neuropathy that affects all sensory modalities. The effect is dose-dependent, occurring at doses of greater than 15mg/kg/day. Both the optic neuritis and neuropathy improve after the medication is discontinued.

Fluoroquinolones

Fluoroquinolones, including levofloxacin (Levaquin®) and ciprofloxacin (Cipro®) have been associated with rare cases of sensory or sensorimotor axonal neuropathy, with painful paresthesias and occasionally weakness. The symptoms persisted after the medications were stopped.

Isoniazid (INH®)

INH® is used in the treatment of tuberculosis. It causes a length-dependent axonal neuropathy by inducing a deficiency of pyridoxine (B_6). The neuropathy is prevented by supplementation with pyridoxine at doses of 10–50 mg a day.

Linezolid (Zyvoxam®)

Linezolid (Zyvoxam®) belongs to a new class of antibiotics (called *oxazolidinones*), which are used in the treatment of infections resistant to antibiotics. Long-term use (over 28 days) has been associated with peripheral neuropathy, and optic neuropathy in some cases. The optic neuropathy may improve after stopping the medications, but the peripheral neuropathy can persist.

Metronidazole (Flagyl®)

Metronidazole is used in the treatment of trichomoniasis or amebiasis infections, and certain anaerobic bacterial infections. In most cases, metronidazole is used for short courses of 7–10 days, but occasionally it is used for long periods in Crohn's disease, or for chronic infections of the bones, joints, or heart. Metronidazole can cause a distal axonal neuropathy after months of treatment, with impairment of all sensory modalities. The neuropathy in most cases is mild, and resolves completely over several months after discontinuing the medication.

Nitrofurantoin

Nitrofurantoin is an antibiotic commonly used for urinary tract infections, occasionally causing neuropathy after chronic use. It can cause a distal axonal neuropathy, with pain and weakness in the hands and feet. Large myelinated axons are preferentially affected. Recovery occurs slowly after discontinuing the medication, but may be incomplete.

Nitrous Oxide (Laughing Gas)

Nitrous oxide gas is used in dental anesthesia, or in combination with general anesthetic agents in general surgery. It causes toxicity by inactivating vitamin B_{12}. People with preexisting B_{12} deficiency can develop complications after a single exposure, but otherwise, chronic repeated exposure is required for neurotoxic effects to occur. Nitrous oxide causes a myelopathy and neuropathy, with damage to both the spinal cord and peripheral nerves. The most common symptoms are numbness and tingling in the arms and legs. In more severe cases, imbalance, weakness, and incoordination can also develop. Improvement occurs after withdrawal of nitrous oxide, and B_{12} supplementation is given to replenish depleted stores. Recovery is generally incomplete.

Nucleoside Analogs ((Zalcitabine (ddC), Stavudine (d4T), Didanosine (ddI))

Nucleoside analogues are used in the treatment of HIV-1 infection. They inhibit reverse transcriptase and prevent viral replication. The neuropathy is dose-dependent, but can begin abruptly. It causes a distal and painful neuropathy, primarily affecting the legs, with impairment of pin and temperature sensations. The neuropathy can progress for several weeks after stopping the medications, and then gradually improve, but with residual deficits. These drugs are thought to inhibit the replication of mitochondria, primarily in the dorsal root ganglia neurons, resulting in damage to the sensory nerves.

Procainamide

Procainamide is used to prevent cardiac arrhythmias. Up to 30 percent of chronically treated patients develop drug-induced lupus. Peripheral neuropathy, which can mimic CIDP, is a rare complication. It presents with proximal and distal weakness, distal large fiber sensory loss, and demyelinating changes, which can be detected by electrodiagnostic studies. This neuropathy is thought to be due to autoimmune mechanisms, and it is treated similarly to CIDP, in addition to stopping the medication.

Phenytoin

Phenytoin is commonly used to treat epilepsy. Chronic phenytoin use has been associated with a mild, distal, predominately sensory neuropathy in the legs. The neuropathy is reversible after discontinuing the medication, with the sensory symptoms improving over a period of several months.

Statins

Statins are commonly used cholesterol lowering agents that reduce the risk of developing cardiovascular disease. Neuropathy, however, has been described in some patients. This neuropathy resolved after cessation of the medication, and recurred after it was reintroduced, confirming the association. Both sensory and motor functions can be affected, with painful sensations, sensory loss, or weakness, in a symmetric or multifocal pattern. Cases of small fiber neuropathy and a syndrome similar to Guillain-Barré have also been described. Statins can also cause myopathy, with muscle cramps and tenderness, and elevated CPK, which can complicate the presentation. Withdrawal of the medication is followed by improvement of both the neuropathy and muscle disease.

Given the widespread use of statins and the relatively high incidence of idiopathic neuropathy, the possibility of statin toxicity is frequently raised when no other cause for neuropathy can be found. There is no specific test for statin neuropathy; but if the condition is suspected, then the medication can be stopped for a period of 3 months to see if there is improvement.

Tacrolimus (FK 506®)

Tacrolimus is used to prevent rejection in organ transplantation. Its use has been associated with both a rapidly progressive axonal neuropathy, and with a progressive multifocal demyelinating neuropathy, with weakness and sensory loss. The mechanism is unclear, but both a direct toxic effect and autoimmunity are suspected. The toxic effects of tacrolimus on the central nervous system include seizures, psychosis, or encephalopathy.

NEUROPATHIES CAUSED BY TOXINS

Neuropathies can be caused by exposure to certain toxins, including heavy metals and various chemicals. These are uncommon causes of neuropathy, except in high risk populations. Most toxins, with lead being an exception, cause a symmetric distal and axonal neuropathy. Exposure usually occurs in industrial or environmental settings where multiple people are affected, providing a clue to the cause. However, some people may be more susceptible to a particular toxin, or the exposure could be restricted, and only one person may be affected. The following is a description of some of the more common toxins that can cause neuropathy.

Heavy Metals

Arsenic Toxicity

Arsenic toxicity most often occurs in industries such as copper or iron smelting, in which arsenic is released as a byproduct. It can occur following chronic low dose exposure, or following ingestion, in which case it is preceded by abdominal pain, vomiting, and diarrhea. Arsenic toxicity causes a distal axonal neuropathy, with pain and sensory loss in the legs and then the hands, followed by weakness after days or weeks. Systemic signs include reddening, darkening, or scaling of the skin, and characteristic changes in the nails, consisting of single transverse white bands, called *Mees lines*. Arsenic is rapidly cleared from the blood, but it remains elevated in urine for weeks or months. It is stored in the hair and nails, and these should be tested if arsenic poisoning is suspected. Higher than normal levels, however, are found in people whose diet is rich in fish, because fish accumulate arsenic from industrial runoff. Treatment consists of chelating agents that bind metals, but because arsenic is rapidly cleared from the blood, the procedure is not always successful, or recovery may occur over months or years.

Other than in the industrial setting, arsenic is difficult to acquire, and accidental exposure is rare. Isolated cases of poisoning are often ascribed to homicide or suicide. Risk factors include substantive wealth and great political power. Napoleon is suspected of having been killed by arsenic poisoning, based on tests posthumously performed on his body.

Lead Neuropathy

Lead toxicity can occur in an industrial setting; following ingestion of contaminated food or drink; or in children who chew objects with lead paint. It can also be absorbed through the lungs or skin. Lead toxicity usually causes neuropathy in adults, but in children it often affects the brain with neuropsychological changes.

Lead neuropathy is unlike other toxic neuropathies because it is mostly motor, with weakness and wasting primarily in the arms and wrists, and less so in the legs. Recent or ongoing exposure can be diagnosed by blood or urine levels, but these are normal in cases in which the exposure occurred years earlier. Lead is stored in bone or teeth, but these are not particularly accessible to testing. Treatment consists of preventing further exposure and chelation therapy, which removes the lead from the body. Improvement is usually gradual.

Lead poisoning is typically associated with other systemic manifestations, such as abdominal pains, impotence, or anemia with small red blood cells. In ancient times, wine was kept in lead containers, and one theory ascribes the fall of the Roman Empire to lead toxicity with associated impotence and neuropsychological changes in the patrician class.

Mercury Toxicity

There are two types of mercury: inorganic and organic. Organic mercury is acquired by ingestion, causing a sensory neuropathy, in addition to visual and hearing loss, and neuropsychiatric changes. Inorganic mercury is usually acquired in the industrial setting by inhalation of mercury vapor, or through the skin. It also causes a sensory neuropathy with psychosis and tremor. Deep sea fish accumulate organic mercury in their bodies, and higher than normal levels are frequently found in people with a diet rich in fish.

Thallium Neuropathy

Thallium is used as a rodent poison and as an industrial agent. Thallium toxicity causes both encephalopathy and neuropathy. The neuropathy is associated with axonal degeneration, and affects the sensory and autonomic systems. It is characterized by unpleasant dysesthesias, sensory loss, and severe autonomic changes. It also causes balding.

Drug Abuse

Inhalation of N-hexane or methyl-N-butyl ketone, which are found in household solvents, fuels, and cleaning agents, can cause a polyneuropathy with axonal degeneration. This most often occurs in teens and young adults.

Other Chemicals

The following chemicals and industrial agents can also cause a predominately sensory or sensorimotor axonal neuropathy:

- Organophosphates, used in insecticides and rodenticides
- Puriminil or vacor, a rat poison that causes diabetes
- Methylbromide, an insecticide that causes pyramidal tract, cerebellar, and peripheral nerve dysfunction
- Triorthocresyl phosphate (Jamaican ginger or jake), a contaminant in illegal liquor or cooking oil
- Dimethylaminopropionitrile, used in the manufacturing of polyurethane foam
- Carbon disulfide (CS2), which is inhaled in industrial settings.

PLEXOPATHIES

Brachial or Lumbosacral Plexitis

Nerve plexus are made up of nerve roots that meet, intercalate, and send out trunks to different parts of the body. The two major plexus are the brachial plexus, which enervates the arms, and the lumbosacral plexus, which supplies nerves to the legs. Injuries result in deficits in the distribution of the nerves that emanate from the plexus. Known causes include trauma, traction, compression or infiltration, radiation injury, and inflammation. Sometimes the cause is unknown, and these cases are considered idiopathic.

Idiopathic brachial plexitis or neuralgic amyotrophy typically begins with severe muscle pain in the shoulder and upper arm. Antecedent events include nonspecific infections, vaccination, or other illness. The pain subsides after 1–2 weeks, but is then followed by weakness in the shoulder and upper arm. Recovery may begin after several months. Most people recover normal function, but there may be residual deficits. In 5 percent of cases, the condition affects both shoulders, although not at the same time. The cause is unknown, but inflammatory mechanisms are suspected, and acute cases are often treated with a short course of prednisone.

Hereditary neuralgic amyotrophy causes a similar syndrome that is inherited in an autosomal dominant fashion. This condition was recently found to be caused by a mutation in a gene called *Septin 9*.

Idiopathic lumbosacral plexitis also begins with pain in one or both thighs and buttocks, followed within a week or two by proximal weakness. The weakness may continue for several months, then stabilize and slowly improve, although often not completely. In some cases, it is associated with significant weight loss. The idiopathic syndrome is similar to that seen in diabetic amyotrophy or following bariatric surgery.

ENTRAPMENT SYNDROMES

Nerves can also be injured by compression, particularly where they course through a narrow passageway that can be further compromised by degenerative changes. Characteristic syndromes are recognized that result from compression of nerves at particular locations with deficits in the distribution of the affected nerves. Subclinical or generalized neuropathies resulting from diabetes, heredity, or other causes can also predispose the nerves to further injury by compression, and this needs to be considered in evaluating anyone with a compressive neuropathy. EMG and nerve conduction studies are particularly useful in identifying the site of compression. The following are some of the more commonly recognized compressive syndromes.

Cervical and Lumbosacral Radiculopathies

Radiculopathies resulting from compression of the nerve roots as they enter or exit the spinal canal most often occur in the neck (cervical) and lower back (lumbosacral), because these areas of the spine act as a hinge and are subject to stress from frequent movement. The sensory or motor roots can be compressed by a herniated disc or a bony spur from arthritis. There is usually pain and muscle spasm over the affected part of the spine, with pain, sensory loss, or weakness in the arm or leg along the distribution of the nerve root that is affected. Electrodiagnostic and MRI studies can help identify the affected nerve root and the cause of compression.

Radicular pain is usually treated with pain medication, in addition to measures that reduce muscle spasm and inflammation, thereby relieving the compression. These include bed rest, muscle relaxants, acupuncture, and nerve blocks that deliver antiinflammatory and pain medications to the inflamed root. If these conservative measures are ineffective, or if weakness develops due to motor root compression, surgery is often recommended to relieve the compression and prevent further damage or development of permanent deficits.

Spinal stenosis occurs as a consequence of compression of the lower spinal cord and nerve roots in the spinal canal. The typical presentation includes *claudication*, which is pain in the buttocks and thighs that occurs after walking for short distances, but which is immediately relieved by stopping or sitting. These same symptoms, however, can be caused by blockage of blood flow to the legs. The latter condition can be diagnosed by Doppler or imaging studies of the arteries in the pelvis and legs. The symptoms of spinal stenosis can be helped by surgical procedures that relieve compression by widening the spinal canal.

Carpal Tunnel Syndrome

Carpal tunnel syndrome results from compression of the median nerve at the wrist. The most common symptom is numbness and paresthesias in the hand or fingers, especially upon waking. Sensory loss in the fingers and weakness of the thumb can also occur in more advanced cases. These symptoms can be aggravated with repetitive movements of the hand, especially if the wrist is held in a flexed or extended position, further compressing the nerve. The diagnosis can be confirmed by EMG and nerve conduction studies. Mild cases can be treated with nonsteroidal antiinflammatory medications and the use of a wrist brace that maintains the hand in a neutral position for at least 2 months, especially at night or during repetitive movements. More resistant cases can be treated with local steroid injections that reduce inflammation. If this is ineffective, and the symptoms are sufficiently bothersome, surgery is often recommended to relieve the compression.

Ulnar Nerve Entrapment at the Elbow

The ulnar nerve lies superficially in the ulnar groove at the medial aspect of the elbow. It is therefore susceptible to direct pressure when leaning on the elbows or flexing and contracting them when moving the arms. Ulnar neuropathy is manifest by numbness and tingling in the last two fingers of the hands. It can also cause atrophy of the first dorsal interosseous muscle between the first finger and thumb, with weakness of handgrip, flexing the fingers, or adducting of the small finger in the affected hand. Therapy using nonsteroidal antiinflammatory agents— and taking measures to prevent compression such as using splints when sleeping—can ameliorate this neuropathy. In more severe cases, surgical intervention with decompression or transposition of the ulnar nerve may provide relief.

Peroneal Nerve Entrapment at the Knee

The peroneal nerve lies superficially to the fibula at the lateral aspect of the knee, where it can be compressed by prolonged sitting on a hard surface, frequent leg crossing, or a Baker's cyst. Compression of the peroneal nerve causes a foot drop, with variable sensory loss along the lateral aspect of the lower calf and back of the foot. Conservative therapy includes avoidance of activities that cause compression and an ankle-foot orthoses for the foot drop. Surgery is only useful if there is an obvious compression that can be relieved.

Tarsal Tunnel Syndrome

Tarsal tunnel syndrome usually presents with burning and shooting pains in one foot, which are worse near the toes. There is often decreased sensation over the anterior two-thirds of the sole, more frequently medially, with sparing of the heel. The tarsal tunnel, which also contains the tibial artery and vein, lies at the ankle on the medial side of the foot. The nerve can be damaged by trauma or compression from tight shoes or casts. Tapping over the tarsal tunnel may induce tingling along the nerve. Conservative treatment consists of removal of any external source of compression, immobilization, nonsteroidal antiin-flammatory agents and medications for pain. Surgical release may be beneficial in more severe cases.

Lateral Femoral Cutaneous Nerve Syndrome

This is a relatively benign syndrome resulting from compression of the lateral cutaneous branch of the femoral nerve by the inguinal ligament in the groin. Compression causes numbness and tingling along the anterolateral aspect of the thigh. Weight loss may help relieve the compression and ameliorate the symptoms.

IDIOPATHIC NEUROPATHIES

In one-quarter to one-third of patients, no cause can be found, and the neuropathy is called "idiopathic." Idiopathic neuropathies are axonal, and may be sensory or sensorimotor. They are classified according to the clinical presentation as idiopathic small fiber neuropathy, or idiopathic large and small fiber neuropathy. Therapy is primarily symptomatic, and directed at relieving the pain and maintaining function with the help of physical therapy.

CHAPTER 6

Management of Neuropathy

THERAPY IN NEUROPATHY is directed at treating the underlying disease, whenever possible, and at ameliorating the symptoms. Treatments for specific causes of neuropathy are discussed under each disorder. The following sections deal with the symptomatic treatments of neuropathy, including pain, autonomic dysfunction, and weakness.

MANAGEMENT OF CHRONIC NEUROPATHIC PAIN

Severe pain can, by itself, be a disease. It can be the most difficult symptom of neuropathy to cope with or treat. It takes over your body and mind; there is no hiding from it and nowhere to escape. It follows you everywhere: to work, to the bathroom, to bed, or when spending time with family and friends. It is hard to think about anything else when you are in pain, regardless of whether you are trying to work, watch a movie, or participate in a conversation. It is like being in a fog or cocoon, with limited interaction with the outside world. Pain colors everything that you do, and can make you depressed, edgy, and seemingly self-absorbed. It can strain your interpersonal relationships, further adding to the sense of isolation and hopelessness that can accompany being sick.

The problem is often compounded by lack of sleep. Painful paresthesias are often the most severe at night, when there are no other distracting sensations. The only thing you can feel is the raging war in your feet. It is hard to fall asleep when your feet are burning or freezing, your body is racked by waves of vibrating or stabbing pains, or the covers feel like sandpaper against your skin. When you do manage to finally fall asleep, you are likely to be awakened after 1 or 2 hours by an even more intense wave of pain. The lack of sleep adds to your physical and emotional exhaustion, and makes it more difficult to function normally or cope with the disease.

Being in pain is a lonely and isolating experience. It is hard for someone who is not familiar with neuropathy to understand how your feet can feel burning and freezing at the same time, or as if stuck with a thousand needles, when there is nothing physically that is obviously wrong. People may think that you are depressed or hysterical, or that you are exaggerating your symptoms. They may not provide much support. People with painful neuropathy often feel alone and with no one to talk to who understands their difficulties.

Depression and anxiety are common consequences of the disease, causing further problems. Treatment of these conditions may not directly affect the pain, but it can affect the consequences of the pain and the ability to cope. The combination of pain, physical and emotional exhaustion, depression, and anxiety can create a downward spiral that is difficult to break. All of these symptoms need to be treated, both separately and together, in order to break the vicious cycle that can make neuropathy such a debilitating disease.

Given the wide array of pain medications and treatments that are available, just about everyone can be helped. However, there is a tendency in our society to suspect anyone who requires chronic pain medication, especially opiates, of being morally suspect or a potential drug abuser. Consequently, many people are undertreated and continue to live with chronic pain. We don't allow torture but the pain of neuropathy can feel the same . Our society needs to understand that pain is an illness needing aggressive treatment, the same as any other disease.

Treatment modalities for pain include oral medications or patches for generalized symptoms, topical medications for localized pain, and interventional procedures when medical management fails. In addition, treatment of depression and anxiety can help a person cope with the disease and limit its deleterious effects.

DRUG THERAPY FOR NEUROPATHIC PAIN

There is no one way to treat neuropathic pain. There are a number of drugs that can help ameliorate the pain, but no one drug works for everyone, and each has different side effects. There is considerable variation between individuals in their response to the therapeutic effect of any particular drug or their ability to tolerate it. The choice of medication is also influenced by coexisting medical conditions and potential drug interactions, which may limit the therapeutic benefit. In general, the drugs used to treat neuropathic pain are effective for all types of neuropathy regardless of the cause, probably because they act on common pain mechanisms.

There are three main classes of drugs that are used to treat neuropathic pain. One group has anticonvulsant (anti-seizure) properties, one has antidepressive effects, and the third, the opiates, are only used for pain. Each group includes multiple drugs that vary somewhat in their efficacy or tolerance in any particular individual. They are frequently used alone, but can also be used in combination because they can have additive or complementary effects. In general, the newer medications in each class offer certain advantages, such as better efficacy with fewer side effects, or longer duration of action, with more even blood levels or less frequent dosing. Given the variability of the individual responses, however, some of the older medications may be beneficial in some patients.

All of the drugs for neuropathic pain have potential side effects, but these occur in a minority of people. When they do occur they are usually reversible by discontinuing or tapering the medication. The process of finding a drug or combination of drugs that provides pain relief without significant side effects is a matter of trial and error, but it is important to recognize what the side effects might be, so the appropriate action can be taken.

The anti-pain effects of the antiepileptic or antidepressive drugs can occur over a wider range of doses than when used for their other indications. However, their use is limited by their side effects at the higher doses. For that reason, the dose is gradually escalated until either a therapeutic effect is achieved or there are side effects. If side effects occur before the therapeutic effect, the medications can be either discontinued or reduced to a tolerable level, at which point another medication can be added in the same manner. If the combination is successful in alleviating the pain, the first medication can then be tapered to see if it is still needed. Alternately, the second medication can be tried after the first is entirely withdrawn, but then a beneficial effect of the combination can be missed.

Too often, beneficial effects are missed, either because the dose is escalated too fast and there are side effects, or because the drug is discontinued before a therapeutic dose is achieved. Of these medications, pregabalin and duloxetine have been approved by the Federal Drug Administration (FDA) for treatment of diabetic neuropathy. Pregabalin, gabapentin, and Lidoderm Patch® are approved for treatment of postherpetic neuralgia. Oxacarbazine is a better tolerated derivative of carbamazepine, which was previously approved for trigeminal neuralgia. Topirimate and lamotrigene are less well tolerated or infrequently used.

Neuropathic Pain Drugs with Anticonvulsant Actions

Pregabalin (Lyrica®)
Begin with 75 or 150 mg/day and increase by 75 mg every 4 days, up to 300 mg/day or 300 mg twice a day. Potential side effects include dizziness, sleepiness, difficulty concentrating, forgetfulness, weight gain, ankle edema, dry mouth, and blurred vision.

Gabapentin (Neurontin®)
Gabapentin is usually started at 300 mg/day and increased by 300 mg every 5 days. A benefit is commonly seen at total doses of 2,700 mg/day or higher, taken in three divided doses. There is little added benefit seen at doses higher than 4,500 mg/day. Side effects include dizziness, sleepiness, unsteadiness, forgetfulness, and fluid gain or ankle edema.

Oxacarbazine (Trileptal®)
Begin with 75 mg at night and increase by 75 mg every 5 days, up to 600 mg twice a day. Side effects include gastrointestinal irregularities, unsteadiness, skin rash, and low serum sodium.

Topiramate (Topomax®)

Begin with 50 mg at night and increase by 50 mg/week, up to 100–400 mg twice a day. Side effects include kidney stones, fatigue, dizziness, memory impairment, word-finding difficulties, anxiety, depression, visual problems, tremor, glaucoma, gastrointestinal pain, poor appetite, and weight loss. Topiramate is removed by the liver and kidneys, and these functions should be tested before its use.

Lamotrigine (Lamictal®)

Begin with 25 mg/day and increase by 25 mg every 5 days, up to 250 mg twice a day. Side effects include a severe rash or Stevens Johnson syndrome, headache, and muscle aches.

Neuropathic Pain Drugs with Antidepressant Activity

Duloxetine (Cymbalta®)

Begin with 30 mg/day and increase by 30 mg every 4 days, up to 60 mg twice a day. Side effects include nausea, dizziness, sleepiness, fatigue, dry mouth, constipation, loss of appetite, excessive sweating, insomnia, and sexual dysfunction.

Amitriptyline (Elavil®)

Begin with 10 or 25 mg after dinner and increase by 10 mg every 3 days, or 25 mg/week, up to 150 mg/day in three divided doses. Helps sleep if taken after dinner. Side effects include drowsiness, dry mouth, arrhythmia, urinary retention, sexual dysfunction, and orthostatic hypotension.

Nortriptyline (Pamelor®)

Begin with 10 or 25 mg after dinner and increase by 10 mg every 3 days, or 25 mg/week, up to 150 mg/day in three divided doses. Nortriptyline has the same side effects as amitriptyline, but with less drowsing effect or postural hypotension. It can be taken in combination: nortriptyline during the day and amitriptyline after dinner.

Venlafaxine (Effexor®)

Begin with 37.5 mg/day and increase by 1 tablet every 4 days, up to 375 mg/day. Side effects include nausea, sleepiness, insomnia, dizziness, headache, hypertension, and sexual dysfunction.

Opiate Use in Neuropathic Pain

Because of their potential for addiction or abuse, opiates are generally used only when other medications are ineffective or cannot be tolerated. If used properly for treatment of pain, however, they can be very safe and effective. In general, the longer-acting formulations are preferred because they provide more even blood levels with fewer fluctuations or breakthrough pain. Methadone has less potential for abuse because it provides pain relief without the euphoric effect of opiates. Shorter-acting opiates, such as tramadol (Ultram®) or codeine, or combinations thereof, are more appropriately used when the pain is occasional or of limited duration.

The following agents have been effective in managing chronic, severe neuropathic pain:

Oxycodone CR (Oxycontin®)
Begin with 10 mg/day; add another 10 mg after an hour if the first dose is ineffective, up to 20 mg every 12 hours or twice a day. Side effects include constipation, nausea, dizziness, and sleepiness.

Fentanyl (Duragesic Transdermal System®)
Apply the patch (25 or 50 mcg/hr) for 72 hours. Side effects include sedation, constipation, respiratory depression, nausea, and low heart rate.

Methadone (Dolophine®)
Begin with 5 mg/day and add 5 mg after an hour if the first dose is ineffective, up to 40 mg/day in 2 or 3 divided doses. Side effects include respiratory depression, sleepiness, constipation, urinary retention, and arrhythmia.

Topical Medications

Lidocaine patch (5 percent)
Lidocaine patches are useful for treatment of localized neuropathic pain, particularly post-herpetic neuralgia. They can be applied for 12 hours at a time to the affected areas. They have few systemic effects

because very little of the lidocaine is absorbed. On occasion, they can elicit a local skin reaction.

Capsaicin (Zostrix® .025 percent, .075 percent)
Capsaicin is the substance in chili peppers that makes your mouth sting. It does so by releasing substance P from the nerve endings. Depletion of substance P prevents subsequent pain. Repeat local applications, at least four times a day, are required so the substance P does not re-accumulate, in which case it can cause stinging after each application. Uneven results have been reported.

Treatment of Muscle Cramps

Muscle cramps, particularly in the calves and at night, are common manifestation of peripheral neuropathy. They almost always respond to quinine sulfate, approximately 300 mg, one or two tablets in the evening. Ringing in the ears or reversible hearing loss are rare side effects.

Treatment of Depression or Anxiety

Several of the medications used for neuropathic pain are also antidepressants, and have added beneficial effects. bupropion SR (Welbutrin®), at doses of 150 mg twice a day, is another antidepressant with some efficacy against neuropathic pain. For anxiety, many patients are helped by clonazepam (Klonopin®), 0.5 or 1 mg per day.

Interventional Therapy for Neuropathic Pain

Interventional therapy for neuropathic pain includes local anesthetic blocks, spinal cord stimulators, and intrathecal pumps that introduce pain medication directly into the spinal canal.

Nerve blocks inject local anesthetics and antiinflammatory agents directly into the painful area: the nerve root, compressive lesion, or sensory or autonomic ganglia that provide pain fibers to the affected region. They provide temporary relief that can break the cycle of pain and reduce muscle spasm. Complications can arise from accidental nicking of the nerve, or if the drug is inadvertently injected into a local blood vessel.

A spinal cord stimulator is usually implanted under the skin in the back, with the electrodes placed next to the spinal cord. It delivers an electric current to the spine, which is perceived as a tingling sensation. The stimulator blocks other pain signals from below, and can be programmed and controlled remotely with an external device. Potential complications include infection, abnormal repositioning, discomfort, and nerve or spinal cord injury.

Intrathecal pumps can be implanted under the skin in order to deliver low doses of pain medications, usually narcotics, continuously and directly to the spinal fluid. This allows for higher concentrations at the target site and avoids systemic side effects. The reservoir is refilled periodically by subcutaneous injection. Potential complications include infection, spinal cord damage, or respiratory depression.

TREATMENT OF AUTONOMIC SYMPTOMS

Orthostatic Hypotension

Treatment of orthostatic hypotension includes both adaptive procedures and pharmacologic agents. Adaptive procedures include standing up slowly to prevent sudden changes in blood pressure, isometric contractions of the muscles while standing or movements such as crossing the legs to reduce pooling, avoiding straining and coughing, which reduce blood return from the legs, increasing sodium and fluid intake, avoiding large meals or alcohol, and putting on elastic stockings before getting out of bed to prevent pooling of blood in the legs.

Pharmacologic agents that help maintain blood pressure include fludrocortisone acetate (Fluorinef®), 0.1 to 1 mg/day, to increase blood volume, and midodrine hydrochloride, 2.5 to 10 mg three times a day, to constrict peripheral blood vessels and increase the flow of blood to the head. A balance needs to be struck between having a sufficiently high blood pressure when standing up, and a pressure that is not too high when lying down. Elevating the head of the bed or using a nitroglycer-ine patch at night can help prevent hypertension while lying in bed.

Gastrointestinal Symptoms

Gastrointestinal symptoms of autonomic neuropathy result from gastro-paresis that can cause bloating or vomiting, and from abnormal bowel motility that can cause constipation and diarrhea. Eating smaller, more frequent meals that have a lower fat content helps reduce symptoms while maintaining proper nutrition. In gastroparesis, domperidone, 10–20 mg, four times a day, and erythromycin 50 mg, three times a day, can lessen the paresis. Constipation is treated with a high fiber diet, increased fluids, stool softeners, and a gentle osmatic laxative, such as lactulose, that prevents absorption of fluid from the gut. Stimulating lax-atives that increase movement of the intestines are usually ineffective and often cause cramping and diarrhea.

Bladder Dysfunction

Bladder dysfunction results from decreased sensation, reduced urine flow, incomplete bladder emptying with retention of urine, overdisten-tion, and overflow incontinence. Milder cases can be helped by frequent and regular voiding. Applying local pressure or contracting the lower abdominal muscles can help empty the bladder. Most people with this condition require self-catheterization several times a day to prevent overflow incontinence. Certain drugs stimulate bladder contraction and are helpful in a some cases; for example, bethanechol, 10–30 mg, three times per day.

Sexual Dysfunction

Autonomic neuropathy can cause erectile dysfunction or ejaculatory failure in men, and failure of lubrication in women. Erectile dysfunction can usually be treated with oral medications such as sildenafil citrate (Viagra®), 50 mg; tadafil (Levitra®), 20 mg; or vardenafil (Nuviva®), 20 mg. However, these agents should not be used by people who have low blood pressure or heart disease because they dilate blood vessels. In women, symptoms can be relieved by the use of estrogen creams and vaginal lubricants.

Abnormal Sweating

Control of sweating by the autonomic nervous system helps maintain a constant body temperature. Increased sweating helps cool the body in warm temperatures, whereas decreased sweating helps the body keep warm in cold weather. In a length-dependent autonomic neuropathy, the ability to sweat is lost in the arms and legs, which are the distal, most affected areas. Compensatory sweating, however, often occurs in the nonaffected areas, such as the chest, neck, or face. Increased sweating can, in some cases, be reduced by glycopyrrolate (Robinul®), trihexyphenidyl (Artane®), or propantheline (Pro-banthene®), although often at doses that are associated with side effects, such as dry mouth, urinary retention, or constipation. There are no medications that stimulate sweating, and care needs to be taken to avoid overheating with physical activity or in hot weather.

ADAPTIVE DEVICES AND PHYSICAL AND OCCUPATIONAL THERAPY

Physical and occupational therapy increases muscle strength and mobility, and helps improve function. This is accomplished through exercising, using braces to support weak limbs or muscles, learning new ways to perform difficult tasks, and learning to use adaptive equipment. Physical therapy does not affect the underlying disease, but helps achieve optimal function within the limitations imposed by the severity of the neuropathy.

Exercising helps improve strength, flexibility, endurance, balance, and coordination. Each of these is accomplished by different types of exercises. In severe cases, overly weak muscles can lead to immobility and contractures, which further reduces strength and limits movement.

A strengthening program, range of motion or stretching exercises, and maintaining the joints in physiologic positions can help improve flexibility, prevent contractures, and increase strength. Therapeutic modalities, such as heat, ultrasound, and massage, can help loosen and mobilize stiff and painful muscles; electrical stimulation can prevent muscle atrophy. Different exercises are recommended, depending on the specific muscles that are affected, the severity of the neuropathy, and the functional impairment.

Adaptive equipment can be used to help overcome functional impairment. Walking canes, crutches, and walkers can help maintain mobility by compensating for weakness or poor balance. Evaluation and training by a physiatrist or physical therapist is recommended for optimal benefit. Other adaptive equipment includes kitchen utensils, toothbrushes, pens, and tools that are lightweight and easy to grip, such as long-handed shoehorns, buttonhooks, special holders for books, page turners, and clothes with Velcro™ closures instead of laces, zippers, or buttons.

Home modifications include raised toilet seats and chairs that make it easier to get up, grab bars in bathrooms and showers, specialized door handles that are easier to grip, hand rails along stairs or corridors, and widened doorways for wheelchair access. Evaluations by physical and occupational therapists are advised for maximum benefit.

Driving can become a problem if you cannot feel your feet, or if you are weak. You might push down on the wrong pedal without realizing it, or not be able to react quickly if a child runs out in front of your car. Installation of hand controls is recommended for safety reasons. Too often, people wait until after an accident or a close call before having these installed.

Caring for Your Feet

Abraham Lincoln was heard to remark, "I can't think when my feet hurt." It is not known whether he suffered from neuropathy, but most people with the disease know that when your feet hurt, it is hard to think about anything else. The feet often bear the brunt of the disease, because the neuropathy is most severe distally, and because they are pressed or pounded by the weight of the body when standing and walking. Hypersensitive feet can be severely painful, and sometimes described as if "walking on a bed of nails" or on "hot coals." Shoes can sometimes make the feet feel as if they are being "squeezed in a vice."

Neuropathy also causes atrophic changes in the skin and loss of thermoregulation, with excessive dryness or sweating. Dryness and dampness contribute to the breakdown of the skin. Dryness can lead to cracking, and dampness increases susceptibility to infection. There may be atrophy of the intrinsic foot muscles, with subsequent loss of protective muscle mass and development of deformities resulting from dorsiflexion (clawing) of the toes, and splaying or widening of the feet on weight bearing. The foot may no longer fit into the same shoes, be more easily traumatized, and be more prone to developing ulcers or pressure sores. The loss of protective sensation can prevent awareness of injury, and treatment may be delayed.

Multiple small fractures in the joints or feet that are allowed to heal without realignment can cause a deformity called *Charcot joint* or *Charcot foot*. Infections, if not treated promptly, can extend to the bone and cause osteomyelitis, in which case amputation may be required to prevent the spread of infection. This occurs more frequently in diabetes, when circulation and immunity are also impaired.

Chronic repeated nerve injury from compression or trauma can cause a condition called *interdigital neuritis* or *Morton's neuroma*. This occurs as a localized enlargement of the nerves, most frequently between the toes, at the 2nd or 3rd interdigital space. It can cause episodic pain, especially when walking. The neuroma can usually be seen by an MRI scan. Treatment consists of injecting steroids and a local anesthetic, or surgical resection.

A number of steps can be taken to prevent or minimize the risk of these complications, including:

1. Avoid high impact activities, such as running, which can traumatize the foot. Participate in low impact exercises such as swimming or cycling instead.

2. Wash the feet daily in warm water, dry them thoroughly, and use moisturizing cream to prevent drying or cracking. Treat excessive sweating with foot powder.
3. Inspect your feet daily for cuts, ulcerations, fissures, pressure sores, blisters, corns, or calluses, and signs of trauma, such as redness or swelling. Seek prompt treatment if any are found.
4. Use a nail file to keep the nails trim and without sharp edges. Avoid sharp instruments, such as scissors or nail clips that might cut the skin; promptly treat ingrown toenails or fungal infections.
5. Avoid going barefoot.
6. If you sprain your foot, make sure you get medical attention because you may need a cast to avoid development of Charcot foot.

It is important to wear comfortable socks and shoes. Use socks made of cotton or wool, without inside seams or elastic bands on top. Shoes should fit properly and be made of soft leather or other materials, also without inside seams. They should leave the toes in a natural position, provide good arch support, and not rub or press against any part of the feet. Cushioning or shock-absorbing insoles can also help reduce the discomfort or pain.

ALTERNATIVE MEDICINES

Alternative medicines include natural products such as vitamins, food supplements, and herbs, or procedures and devices that are believed to be help particular medical conditions or disease. They are different from conventional medications in that their benefits have not been proven by scientific observation or medical experiments. Many people use these to supplement conventional treatments, or when conventional treatments do not work.

Many of today's conventional medications are derived from natural substances that were once considered alterative medicines. Digitalis, for example, came from an ingredient in a witch's brew; penicillin came from bread mold; and Taxol® was discovered in the bark of the yew tree.

Some substances used as alternative medicines, however, have been proven to be ineffective, and occasionally even harmful. Experiments, for example, have shown that garlic does not lower cholesterol as was previously believed, and that excessive doses of vitamin B_6 can cause neuropathy. Megadoses of St. John's wart have recently been reported to produce a painful neuropathy in skin exposed to the sun. The manufacture of alternative medicines is unregulated and their safety cannot be guaranteed. A contaminant in L-tryptophan caused a debilitating condition called *eosinophilic myalgia* several years ago, and some Chinese herbal remedies have been found to be laced with variable amounts of mercury, arsenic, or lead.

Alternative medicines can also be harmful if used instead of proven conventional therapies. One young woman told me about how she and her friend contracted spinal meningitis when they were children. She recovered after being treated with antibiotics, whereas her friend, who was taken to a Voodoo healer, remains paralyzed in a wheelchair. There is a great deal of hype surrounding alternative medicine, without much evidence to support the claims. Lacking experimentation, there is no way of knowing whether a particular alternative medication will turn out to be tomorrow's miracle cure or yesterday's "snake oil."

Proper nutrition, however, is important for the normal functioning of the peripheral nervous system. As discussed earlier, if there is any question about your diet, you can add 500 mg of B_{12}, 50 mg of B_6, 50 mg of B_1, and 400 mg of vitamin E, to make sure you are getting sufficient amounts of these vitamins. If you are found to have a specific nutritional deficiency, such as B_{12} deficiency, then additional supplementation and follow-up blood tests are needed to make sure the deficiency is corrected. If you take multiple pills, make sure the total amount of B_6 is no more than 50 mg daily, because excessive B6 is toxic to the peripheral nerves.

The most common alternative medicines are those used for diabetic neuropathy. These include alpha lipoic acid, at doses of 600–800 mg a day, and evening primrose oil, which contains linolenic acid. Alpha lipoic acid has been reported to help diabetic neuropathy if taken intravenously, but its effect in oral form has not yet been examined.

Other measures, based on trial and error include wearing socks to bed or soaking feet in warm water, if the feet feel cold. Some people reported that applying a solution of wintergreen oil containing dissolved aspirin helped relieve the pain in their feet. These, too, are forms of alternative medicine.

More information about the potential benefits and risks of supplements can be obtained at www.mskcc.org/aboutherbs.

CHAPTER 7

Sharing Stories and Experiences

NEUROPATHY CAN BE A LONELY DISEASE if there is no one to talk to—someone who really understands how you feel, and can help you cope with the physical, psychological, and emotional ramifications. Every person with neuropathy has their own disease, in a way, because neuropathy affects each person's daily routine, work, and interpersonal relations differently. However, anyone with neuropathy can gain strength and hope by sharing experiences and learning from each other. The following stories were written by people with neuropathy, in the hope that their own experiences and thoughts will help others. These stories were excerpted from *Neuropathy News*, with permission from the authors and The Neuropathy Association.

A Nun's Story
Hollywood, The Monastery,
and The Neuropathy Community

R.M. Mother Dolores Hart, O.S.B.

Many times in these past months, I have opened my computer to visit the Neuropathy Bulletin Board on the Internet. I have pondered the numberless accounts of persons with this mysterious disease called "peripheral neuropathy," which now calls me personally into a new community. In my lifetime, I have belonged to two other very different ways: first the community of Hollywood; second the community of the Regina Laudis Monastery; and now, also, the community of those with peripheral neuropathy.

At eighteen, I was signed by Hal Wallis to star in my first motion picture with a young man named Elvis Presley. Of course, I did not experience this as suffering. I was elated, and continued this life, making eleven films in the next seven years and spending a year on Broadway. The films brought me into contact with the greats of those days: Anna Magnani, Tony Quinn, Ernie Kovacs, Robert Ryan, Myrna Loy, Stephen Boyd, Montgomery Clift, Karl Malden, to name a few. As I grew to know the world of Hollywood from the inside, I began to discover that the great actors and actress who seemed to inhabit a world impervious to pain, actually made their roles possible through the transformation of their own inner struggles. Very often their wonderful screen performances were carved out of deep experience of personal pain.

Let me speak of one example everyone knows, Elvis Presley, himself. When I co-starred with him again in "King Creole," our second film together two years later, he had changed a great deal. He was by then a young man in search of himself and wanting very much to take on serious roles. We spoke often on the set about the existence of God and the need to have faith in order to face the ordeal of daily life. I was 20 and he only a few years older. It is hard to imagine now, 40 years later, that even then, with everything before us, the suffering we felt in our own lives took precedence over the enviable pleasure and advantages that surrounded us.

At 24, I entered another community, whose life is more directly concerned with suffering humanity, the Benedictine Abbey of Regina Laudis. An actress is called to present images of the human struggle, no matter how raw, poignant, tender or triumphant. A contemplative community is called to pray for those in the grip of the very same emotions and experiences. We sing the Divine Office in Latin at various hours of the day and night as public form of prayer. In this act of faith, we incorporate the needs of the whole human family in relation to God.

I felt very drawn to the Abbey of Regina Laudis and its effort to live the Rule of St. Benedict as a community consecrated to

God in prayer. Here, where there was a more comprehensive and coherent understanding of suffering, I found that many of the mysteries of my own life, so rich in travels, work, and personal relationships, took on a new meaning and resolution. The act of consecrating my life – body and soul – as a medium for God seemed a natural extension of my dedication to the media of theater and film as a professional actress. And since part of the work of a Contemplative is to personally assume the suffering of a particular people, I felt the monastery gave me a way of maintaining continuity with my friends and co-workers by offering them a new source of stability and strength through prayer. Even though I was not physically present in Hollywood, they knew that, through me, they too had a way to voice their private sufferings and to refuel their energies. My ties with the acting community were not diminished by entering the monastery, but, in fact, continued to grow.

It never occurred to me then that I would once again be put into a totally new orbit of persons. In 1997 after a very serious root canal, I was, of course, not able to eat, but, alarmingly, not able to walk either. That was deep root canal, let me tell you! Two days later, I could not put weight on my feet when I tried to stand. I had previously suffered some trouble with neuromas and grumbled that I had probably upset them by putting too much pressure on the chair during the procedure. It was hardly that simple. Eight months later I was diagnosed with idiopathic sensory peripheral neuropathy.

To find out what to do, I trailed from doctor to doctor, not my own choice, but because the symptom of one thing led to treatment for another, back, bladder, brain and on and on. Of course, each doctor prescribed a pill. The pain in my feet was so constant that I developed TMJ from clenching my teeth at night. The TMJ affected my eating habits and I began to lose weight. Tinnitus sang in my ears, either from medications or from tension. I could not bear the sound of the echo in the church when the Community sang chant, and I even found the quiet of a room unbearable because of the cacophony of ringing and buzzing in my own head.

Right about then, a very trusted physician told me he had discovered I had low thyroid and Hashimoto's Disease [an autoimmune disorder of the thyroid gland]. He was certain this contributed to my neuropathy. He put me on thyroid medicine and told me it would take at least a year. I finally wound up in emergency with hemolytic anemia as a reaction to one of the medications. I remember waking up and thinking, "My God, I can't die now. I just don't feel well enough to meet all those people I haven't seen in so long." Whatever was going on, my immune system was doing its job and the minute the winter flu bug hit the East, I was struck with it full force and developed mycoplasmic pneumonia. Our family physician paid a house call, a rare gift in these days. Though he could not treat the unknown disease of peripheral neuropathy, he said I was a walking pharmacy and HAD to get off so many experimental medications and get some kind of physical therapy as soon as he could get me out of the pneumonia. Soon after, I started exercises in water therapy. All of this when before that darn root canal, I was the picture of health.

The most difficult aspect was the growth of this mysterious and idiopathic (which I now know means "nobody knows") disease and the weird things that were happening inside my own body. When I began talking of the fact that I was walking on nails and felt like my feet were on fire or else I had experienced a "cloven foot," my sisters were quite sympathetic, but God knows what they really thought. The pain developed with all kinds of intricate sidelines, which began to manifest in my ankles and legs. Sometimes I would sit through a conversation when the only thing I really cared about was getting them into a hot bath. The tests of selfless love were endless, as pain grew and became chronic from the moment I got out of bed in the morning.

At one point, my doctors seemed to agree that I had tarsal tunnel syndrome and surgery would be that best thing. But within minutes of setting up the procedure, a phone call came saying to cancel it. A reconsideration of my blood tests and my complaints that I was now experiencing pain in my hips and bladder suggested surgery might not be advisable. So instead, I had a lumbar puncture. The test was easy enough, but need I tell anybody who has had one not to get up too fast afterwards? I did, and felt like I got hit over the head with a sledgehammer. During an attempt to do "a patch," all I can remember is the doctor saying, "Can you handle this?" and then hearing one of my sisters calling me frantically, "Mother, don't go! Count!" *Go where?* I thought, but I couldn't remember what number one was. They rang an emergency bell and two or three attendants came with oxygen and all kinds of equipment. I finally remembered "three" and said feebly, "Can I start with three?" It was awful.

The month passed and I gained strength enough to be sent to a few more doctors, but still the real anguish stemmed from the growing number of signals and shifting places of pain. One day the neuropathy hit my face. The temperature outside was 90 degrees, but I felt like I was wearing an icy mask. My face was cold, not to the touch but from the inside. The nerves in my left cheek would begin twitching and the neurologist who listened to me very sympathetically said in a low voice, "Mother, have you thought about seeing a psychiatrist?"

I went home and wept. Then I got mad. Then I wept again. Then something went through me and I put my hand on the phone to call another neurologist whom I had previously seen. I hit the dial and prayed. He was there and my prayer was answered.

"No, you are not crazy," he assured me. "Write down these symptoms. So many people are being deeply challenged by this disease, but few are told that what they are suffering is real. All suffering is real," he told me, "but local doctors simply don't have the experience when it comes to peripheral neuropathy." He assured me that neuropathy was as frightful as I had imagined. It could travel anywhere in body and cause buzzing and burning, itching, freezing, or shooting pains.

I thought back on moments when I had felt as if someone was ripping my big toe from the second one. How do you describe these things? It took me a while to let myself try because I didn't even want to admit I had something in my body that could not be treated and was advancing in its symptoms. I could feel the nerves in my cheeks jumping and I knew that at a certain hour every day, the freezer door would open and my face would go stone cold until nightfall. Now my fingers were beginning to stiffen. I couldn't the make a fist if I wanted to give a punch! I knew in my heart I feared the next onslaught that might take away a new freedom and that, in itself, gave me reason to believe in devils, even if I had no known theological sources.

Then came the day when I first read The Neuropathy Association Bulletin Board. I took a spiritual leap. There I met other sufferers, many in far worse straits than me. I realized this was now my community, not in a theoretical identification as when we merely call ourselves "one with mankind" and then go about our business. This was my business, like it or not, from moment to moment every day. There would be no escape from being a part of this body of sufferers because chronic pain allows no escape.

I am not easily converted to "religious" answers, in spite of the fact that I am a Roman Catholic convert and a member of a monastic community. I had to find my answers step by step. No doubt this bout with peripheral neuropathy is another cycle in which I must ask, "Why is there pain and suffering in our lives? Why must we reel on a merry-go-round, looking for higher or lower numbers on this test or that, trying this pill or that, and finding ourselves back at the same point months or years later?"

I can only surmise that eventually suffering and pain must become tools that allow for new relationships. No matter what religion we belong to, through submission to the circumstances in which God places us, we can open ourselves to His healing power. And by so doing, discover our own unique mission within the global community that is made up of all of us together.

This is one reason The Neuropathy Association is so important. Through it, we can see at a glance that the burden we carry is somehow mutual, and, overtime, we learn from one another that the very symptoms we share are not simply obstacles to our happiness, but a basis for relationship. Even when there is no actual consistency between the details of our physical experiences, seeing how many others have been engulfed by the reality of this shared disease brings us together in a mysterious bond of brotherhood and sisterhood. After that glimpse into community, no one can go back to accepting isolation.

We do not know how we will beat peripheral neuropathy. It is an avenger attempting to shut us up in a prison to which it appears to hold the lock and key. When I reflected back on my life and then allowed myself to think, "Have I come to this? Am I going to end up being a burden to someone else who must get me this or take me there?" The answer did not come overnight. First, I had to grieve for the "old me" who was now gone, dead. I had to slowly learn the deepest law of spiritual life, which belongs to all religions, and is a key to Benedict's Rule. I had to turn over my very body to someone else, let go and watch another do what I thought was mine to do. The submission it takes to open ourselves is terrible and ultimately the question must be faced: "Will I just center on my own crisis or allow my life to be taken beyond my own center of pain?"

The answer finally did come for me after my talk with my doctor. Indeed, I am now part of a new community, which is inclusive of all that has happened in my life. This new community is made up of you, who are silent redeemers by virtue of the pain you hold, which nobody but you and the few with whom you can share it may even know. I pray that some day the mysterious bond between us will be revealed in all its positive force, but for the moment I know it unites us in a community of hope.

I am grateful to be with you. I have faith that the synergetic power of pain, elevated by each one's option to see the good in the midst of suffering, will help bring about what "old time religion" called miracles!

A Nun's Story: Hollywood, The Monastery and the Neuropathy Community
R.M. Dolores Hart, O.S.B.
Reprinted from Neuropathy News (December 1999) with permission from The Neuropathy Association.

Journey to Health

Andy Griffith

We know you're in impossible pain," the doctor said. "We're here to help you through it." Each of us faces pain, no two ways about it. But I firmly believe that in every situation, no matter how difficult, God extends grace greater than the hardship, and strength and peace of mind that can lead us to a place higher than where we were before. Let me tell you about one of the hardest times in my own life, and how I found this to be true.

I had been alone for a long time when I met an extraordinary woman named Cindi Knight. She had come to Manteo, N.C. to be in a production of *The Lost Colony*, a summer play in which I had got my start several decades before. Our relationship began as a friendship, but as the months passed, I couldn't help but notice her strong faith and gentle strength. Did I mention she was also quite beautiful? Somehow she fell in love with me. Five years after we met as friends, we became husband and wife.

When she married me in April 1983, I was not at the pinnacle of my career. Ageism is rampant in Hollywood, and although I was only in my fifties, work was getting harder and harder to find.

Cindi had had frequent and major attacks of sore throat all of her life. So, shortly after our marriage we returned to Los Angeles and went to see a throat specialist, Dr. Robert Feder. He determined her sore throats were coming from her tonsils, and scheduled an operation. Early the next morning we drove over to the Cedars-Sinai Medical Center and Dr. Feder took out her tonsils. While she was recuperating, I got a bad case of the flu. Not exactly a honeymoon of the rich and famous.

My illness was strange. As I got better, the symptoms of influenza were replaced by pain—terrible, searing pain that ricocheted through my entire body. Cindi and I joked about our invalid status and settled in that Saturday to watch the Kentucky Derby on television. But after the race, when I stood up and took a few steps, I pitched headlong into a nightmare. I was overcome by pain so encompassing that I couldn't feel my feet. I had no control over them, and fell to the floor in agony.

We couldn't reach any of our doctors that weekend. Yet I was so desperate for relief from the pain that I took some of the codeine prescribed for Cindi for her throat. It barely made a difference.

On Monday my doctor met us at a local hospital. There a roomful of doctors attempted to find out what was wrong. For four days they hadn't a clue. Finally they did a spinal tap. When the results came in, one mystery was solved. I had Guillain-Barré syndrome, a rare form of nerve inflammation. It's thought to be caused by an allergic reaction to a viral infection, such as the flu. The nerves become inflamed and begin to send erroneous and scrambled messages to the brain. In some people it causes little pain but extensive paralysis; in cases such as mine, it causes little paralysis but intense pain.

There are no drugs or surgery to treat Guillain-Barré—so the doctor sent me home. "There is nothing we can do," he said. "You've got to ride it out. I'll prescribe some pain medication, but use as little as possible. Come back in a week." The following week he said the same thing. And the week after that. By my next visit I was desperate. If anything, the agony was intensifying. Cindi tried not to let me see her fear, but my physical condition was deteriorating noticeably.

Up to that point we had seen every doctor and specialist I had ever known. Nothing was helping, and the pain had become so consuming that there was nothing else in my life. Then an old friend, Leonard Rosengarten, a psychiatrist, asked if he could come visit. I didn't want a friend to see how bad off I was, so I took my most potent pain medication just before he arrived.

A handsome, white-haired fellow, Dr. Rosengarten had nearly died from cancer of the esophagus, so he knew a thing or two about pain. He pulled up a chair and sat...and sat. He waited until the pain medication wore off and I could no longer hide my agony. Then he went to Cindi. "I know Andy," he said. "He's a stoic if there ever was one. So if he says he's in this much pain, I know he is. Would you mind if I got involved?"

The next morning, true to his word, Dr. Rosengarten got me into Northridge Hospital Medical Center in Northridge, Calif. I was admitted onto an entire floor of people fighting their way back from auto accidents, strokes, and Guillain-Barré. Here, the specialty was therapy and pain management. I'll never forget that day. The doctor assigned to my case brought along a medication specialist. The first thing the doctor said was, "We know you're in impossible pain. We're here to help you through it." At those words, Cindi said she saw my body relax. Just to have the severity of my condition acknowledged was the first step on my journey to wellness. The druggist was there to start me on as much medication as I needed, but then I would be weaned off it as I learned to handle the pain in other ways.

The doctors at Northridge Hospital knew that treating pain meant treating the whole person, not just the body. Everyday we had classes in biofeedback, which taught us how to use our minds to help control the pain. For example, imagining the pain coursing down through your body and out through your toes actually releases endorphins that physically fight pain. But even though my pain was gradually diminishing, my foot still felt lifeless. It was slow going as I shuffled around.

State of mind is crucial, we were taught. Consequently, we patients were all pulling for one another. I'll never forget looking into the dayroom one Saturday and seeing a group of stroke patients in a semicircle, with a therapist behind each of them. The patients were passing a ball from one to another. Each time one successfully maneuvered the ball to the person seated next to him, all the therapists cheered wholeheartedly. There wasn't a bored or blasé staff member among them. It was one of the sweetest and most wonderful scenes I had ever seen.

One day the therapist working on me saw one of my toes move. The whole hospital heard about it. Patient after patient and doctor after doctor stopped by my door and said, "We heard the great news! Congratulations!" I was on the mend.

So instead of lying at home, with nothing to do but dwell on the pain, I was suddenly busy, part of a team, pulling not only for myself but for the others on my floor as well. By the time I left the hospital a month later, I was taking 85 percent less medication than when I arrived. The pain wasn't as severe, and I was equipped to handle it.

Although I was no longer in the acute phase of my illness, we weren't out of the woods yet. It took me nearly a year to recuperate to the point where I could participate in everyday activities. And it was a rough year. My former manager told Cindi and me that we were virtually broke. We thought life would be easier back in my home state of North Carolina, so we put our Los Angeles house up for sale. But the real estate market was bad, and not one good offer was forthcoming.

As I fought my way back from Guillain-Barré, I never stopped thanking God for the help he had provided me through Dr. Rosengarten, but especially through Cindi. Yet I couldn't help but feel bad. She had married me for better or worse and all she had got was the worse.

At the end of that year, I sat in our unsold house with no bank account to speak of and no work in sight. Not only was I old by Hollywood standards, but I had also been out of the game for a year. That alone is hard to overcome. I was getting physically stronger, but I was so depressed. We couldn't sell the house, and I didn't know what to do.

Then Cindi came up with an off-the-wall idea. "Maybe it's a good thing we couldn't sell the house," she said. "Maybe it was God showing us grace. If we moved to North Carolina now you might indeed never work again. What we need to do is stay here and stoke the fire."

That day, and every day for quite a while, Cindi and I went over to The William Morris Agency at lunchtime and sat in the lobby. My agent and every agent in the building saw us. Everybody talked to us, invited us to their offices, some to lunch.

The upshot of it was I got roles in four TV movies that year, including *Return to Mayberry* with Don Knotts and Ron Howard, and the pilot for *Matlock*—a show that ended up running for nine years!

During this period Cindi decided to give up pursuing her own acting career and work with me on mine. I don't know how I would have made it without her.

That was more than a decade ago. Now, though *Matlock* is over, I have a new feature film, and I've recorded an album of my favorite gospel songs. Ageism hasn't left Hollywood, but I hope I'll continue to work.

Guillain-Barré has left me with permanent pain in both feet, but like an unwelcome guest, it isn't so bad when I stop paying attention to it.

Challenges and pain will continue all my life, I know, but with Cindi at my side to remind me to accept God's grace, I'll go forward and continue to work with love and happiness.

Journey to Health
Andy Griffith
"Journey to Health" by Andy Griffith is reprinted with permission from *Guideposts Magazine*. Copyright 1996 by Guideposts, Carmel, New York 10512.

Never Stop Believing in Yourself

Lynn Perlson

I am 34 years old, and one of the most important things I have learned in life is that you have to believe in yourself, even when others doubt you. This is particularly important when you are suffering from a medical disorder like peripheral neuropathy. By far, the hardest thing about this disease was to keep on believing something was wrong with me when my doctors did not. I spent endless hours feeling crazy and misunderstood and even wondering if I was imagining the problem, but I never gave up. Finally, I found a doctor who understood what I was going through and, most importantly, cared. Here is my story.

In January, I had just finished riding my Lifecycle and was talking to a friend on the phone when my leg went numb. I remember telling her that something did not feel right, but I was sure I was just imagining it. Unfortunately, this awkward feeling persisted.

In March of 1992, I met with a neurologist, and thus began my long journey to try to find out what was wrong. I had a battery of tests—you name it, I had it: MRIs to search for brain tumors, multiple sclerosis, EMGs to indicate nerve damage, a spinal tap to rule out God knows what, and more blood tests than I can even list. All the tests came back normal except for one, which revealed a very low level of B_{12}, or pernicious anemia.

The neurologist speculated I might have peripheral neuropathy, but wasn't sure, and more tests were ordered. Meanwhile, my condition was worsening. The numb feeling in my right leg turned into a burning pain which traveled to my arms and hands and eventually everywhere. I felt like someone was taking a blowtorch to my entire body. I loved to walk, but even walking across the street became excruciating. I also enjoyed sports and had played competitive tennis in high school. Unfortunately, due to the pain and fatigue, I could no longer take part in any activity that required use of my legs.

I was given pain medicine, but experienced no relief. Unfortunately, PN nerve pain does not always respond to pain medication. Despite all the different pills I tried, none helped. In fact, they all made me sicker. I couldn't eat. They also gave me double vision, and made me so sleepy I couldn't stay awake at work. And I became so sensitive to light that sometimes just keeping my eyes open was unbearable. I no longer knew what to wear to work, since the burning pain often got so intense I couldn't stand clothes touching my arms. In the middle of winter, I would take my jacket off even though I wore only a sleeveless top beneath it. But that strategy had a catch: the cold air also hurt and made me feel like pins were sticking into me. I was constantly uncomfortable.

On and off through 1995, 1996, and early 1997, I would go back to my neurologist, praying he would finally be able to help me. During this time, one thing did help me tremendously—the Internet. I spent many hours on it trying to better understand what it meant to suffer from peripheral neuropathy. I looked up the side effects of new drugs that were prescribed to me so I would know what could happen before I actually began taking them. Most importantly, I found the Neuropathy Association web page. Because it featured so many stories by and about real people who were suffering with the same disease, it helped me realize that what I was living with was real, too, and that I was not alone.

During the summer of 1997, I finally went to a new neurologist. Unlike other doctors, he took my symptoms seriously. Right from the start, he believed me and never gave up trying to help me. He ordered an EMG and this time, lo and behold, it came back positive. Finally I had true evidence that something was wrong with me. This is what I thought I desperately wanted, but when it actually happened, I was terrified. Now, all of a sudden, I had to face the fact that all of the pain and suffering I lived with was real. And not only might it never go away, it could even get worse.

Because none of the medications I had been taking had worked, my new neurologist decided it was time to get aggressive. He recommended an IVIg treatment called "gammaglobulin." I was extremely hesitant, as it had proven to be successful with autoimmune neuropathy, yet he did not know if that was the kind I had. I consulted my internist, another neurologist, and the Neuropathy Association's web site to learn about other people's experience with the treatment, and then decided to go ahead.

I began the treatment in December 1997 and have had it once a month for the last 8 months. Now, in August 1998, I am happy to say that the treatment has helped. Although I still lose my balance often and get tired extremely easily, I can walk for longer periods. And even though the burning is sometimes so fierce it's difficult, I am undeniably better. Because the treatment has helped, my doctor is now confident that my peripheral neuropathy is autoimmune related, possibly caused by an autoimmune response to a melanoma I had on my right leg in 1989 when I was 25 years old.

Functioning day to day is not easy. Living with neuropathy teaches you very quickly that you cannot take anything for granted. Just a few years ago, if someone had told me that walking up a flight of stairs could be agonizing and make me feel like I'd just climbed Mount Everest, I wouldn't have believed them. Let me tell you: I believe them now.

From the outside, you could never know anything is wrong. I fact, someone recently said how lucky I was that no one can tell I have this disease. Actually, it's a double-edged sword. I don't want people to think something is wrong with me. On the other hand, I often feel like I'm suffering in silence because no one understands what I'm living with. I try very hard to hide what I'm going through. If I lose my balance and fall, I laugh, making people think I tripped. If the burning pain gets really bad and I can't walk, I just pretend I am lazy or tired and let others go ahead. If I can't open my bottle of Snapple, I just plead weakness and let someone else open it for me. Keeping this disease silent takes hard work.

During this entire time, I have managed to work full time in a very stressful industry. I have proven to myself that I can persevere despite tremendous obstacles.

I spent so much time doubting myself and thinking doctors doubted me. But that's over. The most important thing I've learned is to take life one day at a time, never ever give up on yourself, and to keep searching until you find someone who won't give up on helping you. I was so fortunate to have found that in my doctor. I know my life will never be the same, but my doctors, some very special people, and this treatment have given me the most important medicine of all: hope.

Neuropathy, Before and After

Lynn Perlson

When you are diagnosed with peripheral neuropathy, you constantly are confronted with what life was like "before" and "after."

"Before" meant living without having to think about every little thing you do. It meant walking down stairs without having your heart skip a beat as you fear you may tumble down instead of walk down. "Before" meant taking a step without having to take a step.

"After" means thinking before doing. When you wake up in the morning, you get out of bed, remembering to be careful not to lose your balance. You walk to the bathroom to brush your teeth and your legs immediately remind you that you can't take each step for granted. You drink your coffee holding onto the cup for dear life so it won't slip out of your hand. You get dressed knowing that what you put on your body will impact how you will feel for the day. Will the tights you wear with your skirt make your legs burn more? Will the sweater without a layer be a problem if you burn up and can't take it off to minimize the pain? Is the look you're after worth the suffering it might entail?

You change a few times until you're confident you will be as comfortable as possible.

Living with neuropathy means you walk to the subway worrying about falling down the subway stairs. It means riding, in a crowded car, knowing you will have to stand even if standing makes you more physically uncomfortable. If you are lucky and find a seat, you wonder if it is okay to take it as the people around can't see you have neuropathy and may think someone else deserves it more. It means getting to your destination dreading the walk up the stairs. Your eyes scan all the way to the top as your mind continues to tell you "just take it one stop at a time." Ah, you're relieved that you made it, but saddened by the frustrating climb.

You get to work and try and forget about neuropathy and instead think about the work challenges ahead, ignoring for a moment that your morning has already been challenging and it is only 8:45 AM.

Don't get me wrong. You do everything you can to lead as normal a life as possible. No matter how you feel when you wake up, you get out of bed and you go and you never stop going. Yes, you can stop if you need to stop. Yes, you can rest. You can even scream inside because of all the pain. But, you must never think that your life is over "after" you learn you have neuropathy.

It is important to do everything you can to make living with neuropathy a little easier. This includes telling those close to you what you are going through. If you do this, you will learn a great deal about your friends. You will learn that despite the fact that your friends are not living with neuropathy, they can help you to live with it. They can offer to take a cab with you even if they would rather walk. If you do decide to walk, they ask if you're okay. They don't look at you strangely when you lose your balance or grab onto them for support. Most importantly, despite not completely understanding what you live with, they just plain care.

Unfortunately, you will also meet people who don't understand and don't try to understand. So, it is most important that you understand.

Yes, there may be a "before" and "after" to living with neuropathy, but the "after" can be a good thing if you make it that way. You learn to ask for what you need and to take nothing for granted. You even learn to live with the reality of what you have. And if you are lucky, you learn that there are truly special people in this world who accept you for who you are no matter what life is like "after" you get diagnosed.

Never Stop Believing in Yourself
Neuropathy, Before and After
Lynn Perlson
Never Stop Believing in Yourself. Reprinted from *Neuropathy News* (October 1998) with permission from The Neuropathy Association.
Neuropathy, Before and After. Reprinted from *Neuropathy News* (March 1999) with permission from The Neuropathy Association.

How I Spent My Summer in a Blanket

Nancy White

My neuropathy seems to have begun with an injury to my right elbow on April 9, 1996. Tennis elbow, aka tendinitis, was the diagnosis. When I told my orthopedist about the freezing cold and the burning, "electric" tingling in my hand and forearm, he wasn't surprised as those symptoms were consistent with his diagnosis.

The tendonitis improved, but the burning and tingling didn't. Then, one day, I felt the same pain in my *left* arm. And then my left foot and leg. And then my lower back. And finally—and perhaps worst of all—my face. It was summer, which was fortunate, because the colder the temperature, the worse the pain. In fact, if even a gentle summer breeze would blow across my face, it felt as if someone were grinding a lit cigarette into my cheekbones. Air-conditioning was a disaster, which meant no movies, restaurants, or friends' homes. All summer, I dressed in long skirts, socks, long sleeves, high necks, and a scarf over my head and face. I looked as though I was in *purda*, with only my eyes uncovered. For visiting a doctor's air-conditioned office, I wrapped myself from head to toe in a blanket. So, in addition to being in constant pain, I also underwent daily the humiliation of being perceived as, well, just plain crazy. These weren't symptoms with which most people were familiar, or that could easily be explained. Yet they were very real—and horribly, unbearably painful.

Drugs helped. I took heavy-duty painkillers containing codeine, to which I found I was allergic when I broke out in hives all over my body. Occasionally, I took five mgs. of Valium to stop the panic and trembling I experienced when I wondered if this nightmare would ever end. To my surprise, the Valium alleviated the pain for a couple of hours at a time, but, knowing that it is an addictive drug, I saved it for the worst attacks. The burning pain was acute and unrelenting, and I wasn't a brave little soldier. I was unable to work more than two or three hours a day. I cried a lot. I suffered full-blown panic attacks. I considered suicide.

Blood tests for Lyme disease plus those tests we've all had that make you feel like you're being prepared for the electric chair all came back negative. My neurologist suggested I try Neurontin, commonly used to prevent seizures, but also used to control nerve pain. It helped some. Then a second neurologist prescribed Pamelor (nortriptyline), commonly used as an anti-depressant, but again, also effective in controlling nerve pain. He warned me that it might or might not work, and that, in any case, it would be two to four weeks until it would take effect. After just three weeks, it did! I awoke one morning to find the pain dramatically reduced. And after several more weeks, it was virtually gone. I was euphoric!

And now? I'm still taking Neurontin and Pamelor and I still need a Valium once in a while. It's possible that some day I won't need medication. For now, I know I still do, because my hands and feet still feel almost frostbitten when they get just a little cold, and there's still an undercurrent of electric "buzzing" in my hands, especially if they get even the slightest bit chilled. Even after the winter, I wear my mittens when the thermometer dips below 60, and I wear white cotton gloves to work at my computer if my office is drafty. But I'm out of pain, and I have my life back again. And as long as I can say that, I'm not complaining!

How I Spent My Summer in a Blanket
Nancy White
Reprinted from *Neuropathy News* (November 1997) with permission from The Neuropathy Association.

Living with Autonomic Neuropathy

Lizzie Abbot

My husband found me lying on top of a pile of boxes outside of Bloomingdale's. It was not the first time he had gotten a call from me that I couldn't get home on my own. He was used to finding me prone in strange places. We almost had it down to a routine. He would wrap me up in a blanket and take me home. Then, like Peter Rabbit, I would be given a cup of chamomile tea and put to bed. By the time he brought me the tea, I would be out for the duration. Sometimes I slept for 12–14 hours. During this time I would not move or roll over. I would stay so still, my self-winding watch stopped. When my husband would try to wake me, I could not be roused

This was autonomic neuropathy at work. Autonomic neuropathy is a failure in the signals that control our breathing, heart rate, blood pressure and digestive system, those parts of our body over which we have little or no conscious control. Although I had other symptoms, my most dramatic were near faints. I've been known to lie down nearly anywhere, from the bench in the locker room where I swim to the sidewalk. My neuropathy affected my blood pressure. When it dropped, my whole body felt it. If l didn't get enough blood to my head, I couldn't think. I became dopey. I dropped things. I fell down. Sometimes my balance was so affected, I staggered like a drunk. Simple tasks were difficult. Once I sat down on the floor and cried because I couldn't get the key in the lock to my apartment. (I was on the wrong floor.) There were other signs I was losing it. When I put popcorn in a bowl, it ended up on the counter. I fell down on perfectly flat sidewalks, which resulted in a scenic tour of New York City emergency rooms. I couldn't read—my eyes were blurry. I had the attention span of a gnat. Nausea and fatigue were daily companions. My symptoms came and went.

What I hadn't told my husband (and hadn't admitted to myself) was that I often lost control of my bowels and bladder. I learned ways to cope. I kept a complete change of clothes at my office. I was frequently nauseous, and had, upon occasion, even made myself vomit hoping to feel better. Vomiting didn't help, but it did make me sleep for long stretches. Sometimes, afterwards, the nausea stopped.

My first "spell" happened after swimming. I almost passed out going up the pool ladder. I then vomited and had to lie on the bench in the locker room in my wet bathing suit. By the time I was able to get up, my bathing suit was dry. Next time I had a "spell," I was presenting plans for a renovation to a psychiatrist and his wife. He told me to see a doctor.

I didn't have one. My internist and friend of 25 years had retired. In a period of my life filled with losses this turned out to be one of the biggest. We had lost my mother, my father-in-law and my husband's brother, the last through a terrible long death from throat cancer. Each one of us had lost our best friend to other forms of cancer. We moved out of a house we loved because of my problem with the stairs and then we lost our money. Life is a journey, we said. Sometimes there are bumps along the road. We thought we'd handled them pretty well. What we didn't know was that our visit to the land of illness was only the warm-up for the grand tour. That spring, my husband was diagnosed with the same type of throat cancer that his brother had. With a whoosh, our tour bus was off.

Throat cancer is an ordeal. Each phase has its own horror. Behind each one was the shadow of my husband's brother and a feeling that perhaps we couldn't lick it. Our kids were great. We were all trying hard. Without any medical training, I was trying to care for my husband who was barely biologically viable. I was trying to run my job via laptop, e-mail and telephone. I was worn out. My muscles twitched. I had strange electric sensations. Secretly, I thought I was losing my mind. It was stress—I'd read stories about stress. It could play tricks with your mind. I was exhausted—it was depression, no doubt. My husband was depressed. Who wouldn't be?

The psychiatrist on the oncology unit was remarkable. Board Certified in three specialties, he was also the lead writer on the *Manual for Diagnostic Criteria for Mental Illness in the Medically Ill*. We went to see him together. In no time he had my husband on track. One day as he hauled me out of the sofa, he asked what I was doing about my disease. I may have thought I was crazy, but he didn't.

I decided to call the neurologist I had seen a few years before for my burning feet. After a bevy of tests she phoned. "Your test results are back," she said. "You have a degenerative, progressive spinal cord disease. I think it is MS. I'm sorry." I was shocked. I didn't know anything about MS, but I found out fast. MS doesn't have to be, but can be debilitating. She also told me I was a "difficult" case. Before starting MS medication she wanted me to see an MS expert. He agreed with her assessment, but he thought it could also be CIDP (chronic inflammatory demyelinating polyneuropathy). I was relieved that it might not be MS, but concerned that I could not start medication that would slow the progressive nature of my illness. We had to wait for symptoms to develop. Develop they did. My flare-ups were more frequent and severe. Somewhere in here, I decided if l didn't have a diagnosis, my doctors didn't believe I was sick. *I must be crazy*, I thought. I stopped calling my neurologist. When I "crashed" I went to my internist or the ER. After one long, nasty bout, my internist declared with impatience, "You have a serious medical condition! We need to do something." But there was not enough information. I was discouraged. After two and a half years, the MS expert decided I did not have MS. He didn't know what I had.

Just when I was about to give up, I got the information I needed. At my next flare-up, the physician on call was an expert on neuropathy. After some specialized tests, he was able to give me a diagnosis: autonomic and small fiber sensory neuropathy. My falling and dropping things was low blood pressure brought on by a peripheral rather than the central nervous system involvement that would be characteristic of MS.

I am now taking midodrine, which is a miracle drug for hypotension (low blood pressure) even though my neuropathy now includes an abnormal variable heart rate. With the tweaking of various medications, I am feeling better than I ever would have thought possible. Last year at this time I was out of work for eight weeks, barely able to move from my bed to a chair to look out the window. This year, I am packing my watercolor box and brushes to go painting in Tuscany (a secret fantasy). We don't know the cause of my autonomic neuropathy. If it is immune-mediated, there are medications that can make a significant improvement. I am giving myself Enbrel, a powerful antiinflammatory usually prescribed for rheumatoid arthritis. Some people with my symptoms have good results with it. I am hopeful I will be one of them. While I am feeling good now, I can't forget that I have a chronic illness. I need to pace myself.

Some days I believe that my visit to the land of illness has made me a richer, kinder, better person. Sometimes it just feels like a bad trip. But I do have a few tips for fellow travelers. People I expected to rely on vanished, but new friends appeared. I've been surrounded by unexpected love. Coincidences feel like miracles. It gives me comfort to believe they are. Every minute counts. I appreciate where I am today more than ever. My husband is doing well. Each morning when I wake up, I reach out, touch his fingers. I am so glad that we are here, together, today, alive.

Living with Autonomic Neuropathy
Lizzie Abbot
Reprinted from *Neuropathy News* (May 2000) with permission from The Neuropathy Association.

Peripheral Neuropathy: Can This Disease Be Stomped Out?

Marguerite "Mims" Cushing

It is 6:45 a.m. in Ponte Vedra Beach, on a barrier island in north Florida, my home. Tropical plants brush my legs as I walk along the pathway on this roasting day in August. The resident alligator is taking a sunbath near the lake. Walkers, bikers, runners nod to me and pass by swiftly. Jerry, a neighbor, tips his cap and pounds past, running along Creekside Trail in the opposite direction. "Hey, How are ya? Ya got that serious walk today!" You're damn right, Jerry. Yes, I've got that serious walk. I am pounding my feet into the concrete. I am angry at them.

During the course of the day if I try to sit and rest with my feet up, it feels as though electrical currents are coursing through each foot, that my toes are plugged into an electrical outlet. At night I'm sure 1,000 ants are wiggling to be free. Sometimes my feet pulsate or feel as though they're fireballs, ready to explode. There's a submarine in there, pinging its heart out. It feels like the worst imaginable sunburn.

I have a condition called "peripheral neuropathy," which means in its simplest definition, damage to peripheral nerve endings, usually irreversible. Early on I didn't know about the irreversible part, I just thought it was a temporary thing—as in, it's no big deal; it'll stop soon.

I look down at my feet and alternate between barking at them, "Are you out of your mind behaving like that? Quit it, you brats!" and mollycoddling them, cheerleading: "It could be worse, little piggies. Get better!"

If you look at my feet they don't seem abnormal. No bruising, no bleeding. No swelling. It feels as if they're double their normal size. I must be wearing a thick sock or shoe, I tell myself when I lie down, and then I remember—no, it's the neuropathy. People have been known to climb into bed with their shoes on because they can't tell if they're on or off. Sometimes I think my eight-pound poodle, Charlie, is lying on my feet and I try to whoosh him off the bed—but he's by the window, dreaming of conquering 'gators.

One Day in January

My "little problem" started in January of 1996, right after my 52nd birthday. I can divide my life into two parts: before PN, and after. My husband and I drove, sunroof open, jazz blaring, to a new mall in Georgia. It was a chilly, sunny Sunday, the type of winter day northern transplants call "the reason we moved to Florida." I found a store that sold deck shoes, and bought a pair, the first ones I'd ever owned. I wore them for a couple of weeks. My feet started to burn and tingle. *Phooey, I'm allergic to the shoes*, I thought, and threw the expensive things in the back of my closet. The tingling, burning continued.

I bought a small whirlpool footbath, which soon turned into a drinking bowl for the dog. My nerve endings had gone haywire: cold water made my feet feel as though they were freezing. Hot water was out of the question— it made my soles burn more. Tepid water? Useless.

About a month later, any shoes were driving me wild. To ease the burning, I wore socks with flats or sandals. Not a pretty fashion statement. Putting on the softest socks was like pulling sandpaper along the soles of my feet. In bed I couldn't bear the weight of a sheet or blanket. The best sensation was (and is) cool wood floors. But not cold tile. Brr!

Many weeks later, I went to my internist. My deck shoes were not the problem. Because she knew one-third of neuropathy sufferers have diabetes, she checked me for that, but results came back normal. I didn't realize how lucky I was: most people go to doctor after doctor until they are correctly diagnosed. She suggested a neurologist. I was dumbfounded. No one in my family had ever needed one.

Surely there's a pill somewhere...
Reluctantly, I did make an appointment with a neurologist, still thinking I should let time pass and the problem would fade. On my way to see him, even with the A/C blasting, it felt as though a furnace was raging near the pedals. When I put my fingers near my calves to "feel the heat" my hand felt only the cool air. I remember thinking, *If I tell the doctor this, he'll think 'this woman is a nut case'.*

The neurologist ordered tests including an EMG—electromyography—to measure the electrical properties of the nerves. The results were negative, proving that I didn't have certain diseases. But those early tests didn't prove that I did or did not have neuropathy either. The doctor guessed I had some kind of sensory neuropathy. He implied there was nothing he could do. "I'm sorry about your pain," he said, even though I'd told him I couldn't describe what I had as pain. "Pain," I said to him, "is childbirth. This is not childbirth."

Whoever heard of such a weird disease?
I started devouring information about peripheral neuropathy and found more than 100 different reasons why a person can have neuropathy, such charmers as Lyme disease, thyroid problems, alcoholism, AIDS, cancer, rheumatoid arthritis, kidney disease, and on and on, even leprosy. I asked every doctor I came in contact with about neuropathy. A podiatrist said he sees five or six people each week who complain of the same problem What a complicated disease! One person's symptoms may be entirely different from another's. And symptoms change day to day.

But the annoyance escalated and finally in January of: '99, I discovered a website, that led me to a doctor who is a leading researcher of the disease. I made an appointment with him. He found I had numbness, loss of sensation, and loss of balance. After taking 16 vials of blood and doing quantitative sensory testing (QST), he determined that my neuropathy's etiology is unknown, as in "idiopathic" which to me sounds like a combination of idiot and pathetic.

The doctor prescribed Neurontin, used today for neuropathy sufferers. It is a drug whose label use is to help epileptics, a fact that I found bizarre and scary. Today I just feel...hey, whatever. It does lessen symptoms.

I learned that The Neuropathy Association has estimated over twenty million people in the U.S. may have the disease. Some don't know they have it because they're in the early stages. Peripheral neuropathy is in most instances, not life-threatening, but many people must go on disability because of chronic pain.

I became used to blank stares from friends when describing the symptoms. Their look said, "What are you talking about?" They asked, "If your feet are numb how can you feel the burning, stabbing, and tingling?

I told them that my feet are like the United States: there can be a blizzard in Boston, sunshine in Miami and a tornado in New Orleans.

I wanted so badly to go to a support group and wished Jacksonville had one. So, I decided to form one, not knowing how. The Association gave me a lot of assistance. At our first gathering in October 1999, six people showed up at our hospital meeting room. An hour into the session, we found one attendee had come upon us while trolling the corridors, having tired of visiting her husband, recuperating from a heart attack. We jumped from six people to thirty at the second meeting. In less than two years, my index box indicates almost 200 people have come to our meetings, of which several dozen are regulars. We are family.

Toughing it out is not the way to go

It's perfectly understandable that friends think we who have the disease are exaggerating. ("Oh yes, I know. My feet get hot too.") Or they think excess weight is the culprit. But I find it inexcusable that some doctors are so poorly educated about it. They tell patients. "You have to live with it." A respected internist in Stamford, CT told me "Just forget about it." As it turns out, forgetting about it is the worst thing you can do. Shame on all of those doctors! It's a bad idea to use the tough-it-out philosophy. The longer you wait to seek help, the harder it is to control. Eventually you do have to get on with your life, but you need to establish a baseline and get medication to calm things down, if possible. Many people find lotions and moisture creams can soothe their feet at night.

The hardest thing about peripheral neuropathy is trying to explain it to loved ones. My daughter and I had blissful moments after her first child was born. But now my three granddaughters are under the age of four and I'm not able to play the way I want to. The Neurontin saps my energy. It is joyous to monkey with the kids at a park, though I usually pay for it with a flare-up at night. The sheer delight of playing takes my mind off the feet gremlins most of the time.

Someday a cure will come

It is 7:30 a.m. I've been walking for forty-five minutes to a tape of polkas. Tomorrow, I'll switch to parade music. Humidity exacerbates the neuropathy problem and makes prickly sensations go up to my knees or thighs. Summers are difficult in Florida. We are the lightning capital of the world. TV bombards us to take cover and crouch low if we feel a tingly, electrical sensation in our feet. I just laugh, because the electricity is my nearly constant companion.

Summer or winter, walking 40 minutes first thing in the morning helps. Does the energy boost give me a natural high? Probably. Does it help the circulation? Maybe. Do I feel better just doing something that's positive physically? Absolutely. But I never know how much I'll be able to do. Sometimes, by midday, this shopaholic can only walk for a short time at a mall. Other days, I can stay there as long as I want. I'm grateful my car has cruise control so my hands—just beginning to be affected—can do much of the accelerating and decelerating. Actually, I'm grateful that I don't have the dozens of diseases du jour that are mushrooming all over the country.

For now, the best symptom-relieving "pills" for many people are the little support groups that chug along month after month, gathering steam, gathering passengers, and spreading word about peripheral neuropathy.

Peripheral Neuropathy: Can this Disease Be Stomped Out?
Marguerite "Mims" Cushing
Reprinted from *Neuropathy News* (December 2001) with permission from
  The Neuropathy Association.

Peripheral Neuropathy in Your 80's, A Personal Story

Bertram Schaffner, MD

It never occurred to me that I would ever have trouble with my legs or walking. My legs had always been such a dependable and natural part of me. When I was a very young child, my grandfather used to get pleasure from having me "dance" and would reward me with a bright shiny dime. I really enjoyed long hikes, swimming, climbing mountains, and of all the sports, I preferred tennis. People told me that they liked the way I walked. I also walked very fast, with long strides, and I had endurance.

So it hit me very hard when, at the age of 86, I noticed that I was walking "strange." I had no idea whether this was due to difficulty in my nerves, bones or brain. I only knew that I seemed to lurch to the left from time to time while walking along the street, and that I had no control over these sudden losses of balance. I thought it might look to people as though I was staggering while drunk; I couldn't understand what was going on. My feet did not feel "real" to me; they felt as though I were wearing heavy socks, and as if they were weightless. My sensitivity to pinpricks and vibration was greatly diminished.

I first consulted two neurologists with excellent reputations, one of whom told me that I was just suffering a symptom of old age, and should try to get used to it. The other one seemed very skeptical about what I told him.

A third neurologist, to whom I am grateful, identified my problem as a form of peripheral neuropathy. I burst into tears as I realized that my carefree days of enjoying being on my feet without a second thought were over. However, his diagnosis freed me to begin to explore and study the nature of my condition. It turned out to be extremely difficult to find anyone who could shed more light on my particular symptoms or how to treat them.

I learned that two doctors, one in London and the other in Australia, were using infusions of immunoglobulin and that they were reporting some favorable results. I telephoned each of them to arrange a consultation. The Australian doctor happened to be in the United States for a conference on peripheral neuropathy, but was leaving that same day for home, and I was not ready to make a trip to Australia at that same moment, so I decided to try to contact the Londoner. He was on his way home from the same conference. We made an appointment, which he had to cancel at the last minute, when he was called to Israel on an urgent mission. However, he told me that fortunately there was a doctor in New York who might be able to treat me. This new doctor sent me for tests, which revealed that I had a type of neuropathy called "CIDP," or "chronic inflammatory demyelinating polyneuropathy." Treatment began with biweekly intravenous infusions of immunoglobulin and has continued ever since.

I began to get better. First, my feet started to feel "real" again, and I was more sure of their location when I was walking. They also felt more solid. Unfortunately my sense of equilibrium has never recovered, and therefore, to be sure of maintaining my balance, I have learned to steady myself with a cane when I walk outdoors. Much better than looking drunk! At home, I have arranged the furniture in such a way that I do not need a cane, there is always something near on which I can lean, if necessary. Using a cane has a tendency to make one lean to one side, and I have learned to counteract that by carrying something with a little weight in my other hand. I discovered that I feel more secure when walking near a wall away from the curbside of the sidewalk, where there is nothing to lean on. I feel safest of all when holding onto a railing, or running my elbow along the wall to provide the cues that enable my body to stay upright. I came to understand that my lurching had a lot do with missing the sensory cues from my feet that would have informed my sense of balance. I also felt better because I can now understand my symptoms more fully and take steps (no pun intended) to prevent them.

Another doctor pointed out that I needed instruction in walking! I never dreamt that one's walking could be incorrect. I consulted a personal trainer for help with body movements. He and his assistant have been invaluable to me. While the trainer emphasized stretching and muscle strengthening, his assistant concentrated on locating and reactivating muscles that I was not using. She has taught me the sequence of movements in walking that I was unaware of, and improved my understanding of what is involved in attaining good functional posture. I am especially grateful to her for teaching me how to breathe properly. I had no conception of its importance until I began working with her. I now have the mental concentration and muscular control I need to keep from lurching.

I am no longer as depressed or pessimistic about my condition. I seem to have taken it in stride (again, no pun intended). I automatically remember that it takes me longer to get somewhere than it used to. I have accepted the fact that I cannot walk long distances. This was quite a problem at first, since I have loved visits to museums requiring long periods on my feet. I have made peace with using a wheelchair in these special circumstances, and accept gratefully the offers of friends to wheel me around. Best of all, I am able to enjoy much of my regular life, even including navigating airports and travel.

So, if you are in your 80s and are told that the reason you can't walk is because of old age, or that you can't be treated, don't listen. See your neurologist and show him or her this article.

Peripheral Neuropathy in Your 80s: A Personal Story
Bertram Schaffner, M.D.
Reprinted from *Neuropathy News* (December 2002) with permission from
   The Neuropathy Association.

From Almost Total Muscle Failure to Functioning Again. It's Almost Like a Miracle!

Augusta Dellimore

Before October, 2000, I was a healthy, happy, energetic 50-year-plus young woman. Or so I thought! So what happened? How did go from a seemingly perfectly healthy individual to almost dying from respiratory failure?

In October, I was on my way home from the gym when I noticed a very light tingling sensation in my fingertips. I dismissed it as inconsequential; perhaps I had squeezed the weights too tightly. In November, I saw several doctors, but they could find nothing wrong. My condition grew progressively worse. The tingling had intensified and had moved down into the palms of my hands. I began to have a myriad of other sensations in my hands: extreme burning, throbbing, numbness and weakness. I had no grip. Things started falling out of my hands, which felt swollen and inflamed as if they were constantly on fire.

Flash forward to April, which was not a good month, although the worst was yet to come. All the sensations I was having in my hands traveled down to my toes and the soles of my feet. "What's going on?" I kept asking myself. My body was spiraling downhill, and after a multitude of tests, doctors still did not know what was wrong with me.

In May, I began to have weakness in my elbows and shoulders. I could not lift my arms. They felt as if they were locked. I had to call Fatima, my neighbor and friend, to help me. I had always been such an independent person. I loved helping others, but never really needed this kind of assistance myself. Things were fast mushrooming out of control. I went to the Emergency Room, but they could find nothing wrong.

Later that month, I was scheduled to have another EMG at the hospital. By then, I was having so much difficulty walking and with movement in general, I was afraid I wasn't going to be able to get there. I'm a stickler for punctuality, but arrived a half hour late. While I was lying on the table, I became aware of someone standing over my head, looking in the direction of the computer. After a while, he introduced himself. His words were few: " I think I know what your problem is." Can you imagine the excitement I felt at that moment! After "doctor hopping" for more than seven months, finally, someone had an idea of what was wrong with me. And not a moment too soon!

He explained I had a condition called "CIDP." For reasons as yet unknown, the myelin sheath (the protective coating on the peripheral nerves) becomes damaged or destroyed. He said my case was one of the worst he'd ever seen, and told me about the different types of treatment for this condition. How elated and relieved I was! Someone had finally diagnosed my condition, and knew how to treat it!

In the meantime, my body continued on its downward spiral. In fact, it had almost ceased to function. I was unable to walk a couple of times; I fell down in my apartment and needed someone to help me get up. I could hardly use my hands. My voice was fast disappearing. I began to have difficulty breathing. I soon realized that if I were unable to speak or write, I couldn't communicate. I was in real trouble. I made an emergency call to my doctor who arranged for a nurse to come to my home and administer one of the treatments he had told me about: intravenous gammaglobulin, or IVIg.

The treatments were given for five days. On the second day after the IVIg, I was able to lift my body just a little although my balance was still precarious. I rocked backward and forward. However, I was able to walk or should I say "bounce" around the apartment a little bit. My legs felt as if they were made of rubber. By the third day, I was feeling much stronger. I was still rocking and tilting, but I was actually able to walk three long blocks to the post office to pick up my mail. I was able to lift my arms from their locked position. I was even able to use my hands again. It was like a miracle—I went from almost total muscle failure to functioning again in just three days! The following month, I received the treatment again for five days.

Since then, I've tried to help myself by learning everything I could about this horribly debilitating condition. I've found some very enlightening on the Internet and from books in the library. I have included in my diet food supplements like flaxseed oil, the essential fatty acids (EPA and DHA) and lecithin. I have learned from my research that these substances assist in the rebuilding of the myelin sheath and help support the integrity of the peripheral nervous system. It is now seven months since I started treatments for CIDP and I'm happy to report that I feel great! Once in a while, I'll still feel a little burning sensation on the soles of my feet and some tingling here and there, but I know my body is still going through the healing process. I believe that what helped me to persevere through the ordeal until help arrived was my positive mental attitude and faith in God. I believe it was the working of a Higher Power. And that's why I call my doctor my "Angel." To those of you afflicted with CIDP, I say there is hope for a better tomorrow. My prayer is that you, too, will find your "Angel."

From Almost Total Muscle Failure to Functioning Again. It's Almost Like a Miracle!
Augusta Dellimore

Reprinted from *Neuropathy News* (June 2002) with permission from The Neuropathy Association.

Resources

PATIENT ORGANIZATIONS

The Neuropathy Association

Provides support and education, advocates for patients' rights and access to care, and funds research into the causes and treatment of peripheral neuropathy.

www.neuropathy.org

Tel: 212-692-0662

The Charcot-Marie-Tooth Association (CMTA)

Dedicated to improving the quality of life for people affected by CMT disease.

www.charcot-marie-tooth.org

Tel: 610-499-9264

The Guillain-Barré Syndrome International

Provides informative support and opportunities for patients, families, and friends to network and cooperate.

www.gbsfi.com

Tel: 610-667-0131

RESEARCH INFORMATION

The National Institute of Neurological Disorders and Stroke

www.ninds.nih.gov/disorders/stroke

INFORMATION REGARDING HEALTH CARE PLANS AND PAYMENT ASSISTANCE

Patient Services Incorporated (PSI) is a non-profit organization that specializes in co-payment waiver assistance for people with chronic illnesses.
www.uneedpsi.org
Tel: 800-366-7741

The National Committee for Quality Assurance provides free access to detailed report cards on health plans, clinical performance, member satisfaction, access to care, and overall quality on its Health Plan Report Cards Online.
www.ncqa.org

BOOKS ON NEUROPATHY AND COPING WITH CHRONIC ILLNESS

Baier, Sue. *Bed Number Ten*, CRC Press, Houston, TX, 1989.
Tells the story of a patient totally paralyzed with Guillain-Barré syndrome.

Caudill, Margaret A. *Managing Pain Before it Manages You* , The Guilford Press, N.Y., N.Y., 1994.
Provides practical approaches to help cope with daily pain.

Cole, Jonathan. *Pride and the Daily Marathon*, MIT Press, Boston, MA, 1995.
A gripping story of how one man overcame a debilitating sensory neuropathy that left him without sensation.

Cousins, Norman. *Anatomy of an Illness*, Bantam Press, N.Y., N.Y., 1991.
This book is about overcoming illness and the human spirit.

Cushing, Mims. *If you're having a Crummy Day, Brush Off the Crumbs!*, Mims Chushing, Ponte Verde Beach, FL, 2002.
Offers neuropathy sufferers ways to get through particularly bad days.

Senneff, John. *Numb Toes and Aching Soles*, MedPress, San Antonio, TX, 1999.
A layperson's guide to the peripheral neuropathies.

Wheeler, Eugenia G. *Living Creatively with Chronic Illness: Developing Skills for Transcending the Loss, Pain and Frustration*, Pathfinder Publishing, CA 1989.
A self-help book for people who are chronically ill, and their families, friends, and caregivers.

Index